HELP FOR WORRIED KIDS

How Your Child Can Conquer Anxiety and Fear

CYNTHIA G. LAST, PhD

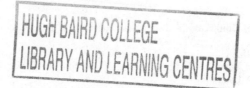

THE GUILFORD PRESS
New York   London

© 2006 Cynthia G. Last
Published by The Guilford Press
A Division of Guilford Publications, Inc.
72 Spring Street, New York, NY 10012
www.guilford.com

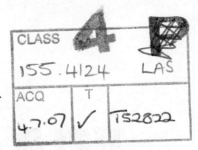
The information in this volume is not intended as a substitute for
consultation with health care professionals. Each individual's health
concerns should be evaluated by a qualified professional.

Printed in the United States of America

This book is printed on acid-free paper.

Last digit is print number: 9   8   7   6   5   4   3   2   1

Library of Congress Cataloging-in-Publication Data

Last, Cynthia G.
   Help for worried kids : how your child can conquer anxiety and fear /
Cynthia G. Last.
       p.   cm.
   Includes bibliographical references and index.
   ISBN 1-57230-858-3 (trade paper) — ISBN 1-59385-219-3 (trade cloth)
   1. Anxiety in children—Popular works.   2. Anxiety in children—
Treatment—Popular works.   I. Title.
   RJ506.A58L37 2006
   618.92′8522—dc22
                                                    2005014040

HELP FOR WORRIED KIDS

To all the little ones I met along the way

Contents

viii   Contents

Acknowledgments

There are many people to thank when completing a book like this. I first want to acknowledge the mentors and colleagues who played pivotal roles in the development of my career: David H. Barlow, PhD; Michel Hersen, PhD; the late Joaquim Puig-Antich, MD; David Kupfer, MD; and Frank DePiano, PhD.

I also want to thank the administration of the National Institute of Mental Health for affording me so many opportunities to investigate and learn more about anxiety disorders in children.

I want to express my appreciation to Kim Sterner, who worked by my side for over fifteen years, first at the University of Pittsburgh School of Medicine and then later on at Nova Southeastern University in Florida.

Special thanks are due to my editors, Kitty Moore and Christine Benton, as well as the staff at The Guilford Press, for making this book a reality.

I am grateful to my husband, Barry Rubin, for supporting and encouraging me throughout the writing process, especially when times got tough.

Finally, I will always be indebted to the many children and families I've had the privilege to meet and work with throughout the years. They are the true inspiration for this book.

Preface

Although it's hard to believe that time has passed so quickly, I realize that I've worked with anxious children and their families now for nearly a quarter of a century. The work has taken several different forms—as director of university-based clinics for children and adolescents with anxiety disorders, as investigator on numerous research grants and scientific studies that focused on understanding and treating these conditions in kids, and last, but by no means least, as a practitioner. Over the years I think it's safe to say that I've seen literally thousands of kids with these problems.

There's no question that this wealth of experience has played an enormous role in the writing of this book, but there is another experience—one of a more personal nature—that gives me an additional perspective on worries, fears, and anxiety in young children. I was one of these kids. But at that time, in the late fifties and sixties when I was growing up, there was "no such thing" as anxiety disorders in children. My parents, pediatrician, teachers, and camp counselors—all witnesses to my overly anxious ways—considered it a temporary phase, one that I eventually would grow out of.

But they were wrong. While kids "grow out of" *normal* worries—like fears of monsters or thunderstorms when they're five—they don't grow out of more serious forms of anxiety. In fact the opposite usually happens—they get worse as they get older.

When I was starting out in my career, there was a lot happening in the professional community for *adult* anxiety disorders but virtually nothing for kids who had these problems. When we opened the doors to the Child and Adolescent Anxiety Disorder Clinic at the University of Pittsburgh School of Medicine in the mid-1980s, to the best of my knowledge it was the first program of its kind. And when I received my very first research grant from the National Institute of Mental Health around the same time—to study "childhood anxiety disorders"—that too was entering new terrain.

Today, decades later, things are different (I'd like to think in part due to the attention I brought to this area). There are numerous programs and centers that specialize in assessing, diagnosing, and treating childhood anxiety disorders—not just in the United States, but all over the world (see the Resources section of this book for the locations of some of them). There have been dozens of research grants and hundreds of studies of anxious children so that we now know a tremendous amount about how anxiety disorders manifest themselves in kids and how they're best treated.

Although the medical and mental health communities have benefited from this accumulated knowledge, it has been shared in a very limited way with parents. Television programs and magazine articles can give only a brief glimpse into the experience of anxiety in kids and very rarely deal with how you—the parent of an anxious child—can help your son or daughter get past the problem.

And that, in a nutshell, is my reason for writing this book. To share with you all that we know about kids like yours and, especially, to give you specific practical and powerful steps you and your child can take *right now* to turn things around.

Regardless of what your child is worried about, this book tells you what the two of you can do so your child will worry no more. And by taking charge and conquering the problem early on—while your child is still in elementary school—you'll not only be making things better for him or her (and your family) now; you will, in all likelihood, be giving your child a better future.

PART I

Understanding Your Anxious Child

1 DO YOU HAVE AN ANXIOUS CHILD?

Michelle's parents don't know what to do. Their daughter is afraid of a lot of different things. She shakes when she sees the neighbor's dog, she's nervous about sleeping in her own room, and she's anxious when she's in a new situation—like the first day of the school year, starting day camp, or going away with her family on vacation.

Michelle's pediatrician says it's just a stage she's going through—that she'll "grow out of it" when she gets older. But her parents know they didn't go through this with her older sister. And Michelle's friends don't act like her.

How can they be sure what Michelle's going through really is normal? Or does she have a problem they need to pay attention to?

The elementary school years can be a stressful time for parents. Your child, who was "your baby," is now a little person.

During this period, children change in many ways. It can be hard to know whether what you're seeing is a normal phase that all kids go through or a sign that your child has a problem, something you need to give special attention to.

Children experience many fears and anxieties as part of their normal development. In some cases, though, these fears and anxieties go "beyond normal" and interfere with your child's well-being.

If you're reading this book, you probably suspect there is a problem. Maybe you've observed that your son or daughter is more fearful than his or her friends or the other children in your family. Maybe your child's doctor, teacher, or even a mental health care professional has said that your child is overly anxious.

To know for sure whether there is an anxiety problem, you first need to be aware of exactly what *is* normal. Which fears and anxieties are expected—are considered normal—during a child's development?

> **Before you can determine whether your child has an anxiety problem, you need to know which fears and anxieties are part of normal development.**

The Normal Fears of Childhood

The objects and situations that children fear most probably are not sources of anxiety to you, and it may be hard to fathom how harmless things—like thunderstorms, unfamiliar people, or a dark room—can cause your child so much distress. If this is your first child and you have not been through this before, this is particularly understandable.

All children have fears. The so-called "normal" fears of childhood are referred to as such because they occur, almost without exception, among all boys and girls—in children from all races, nationalities, religions, and ethnic groups, and among families with different financial and living situations.

Each of the common fears of childhood is linked to a particular age period. I've listed the usual ages of onset for them in the sidebar on page 5. For example, before your child is two you will see a number of fears appear, including "stranger anxiety" (fear of unfamiliar persons), separation anxiety, fear of high places, and fear of loud noises and looming objects. These fears may continue for several years, even up to the age of five. The way they look, however, changes as your child gets older.

Let's use separation anxiety as an example. Billy, who is eighteen months old, shows his fear of separation by screaming and turning red in the face when his mom leaves the room. Clara, who has just entered kindergarten, shows her separation anxiety differently, in a way that's more appropriate to her age. For the first few days of school—until she's familiar and comfortable with her new surroundings and being away from her home and mother—Clara pleads with her mom to let her stay home.

When children are a little older, at two or three years of age, fears of the dark and small animals develop. Fear of the dark can continue for quite some time, even up to age seven or eight. Seven-year-old Tyler insists on having a nightlight in his bedroom and having the door to his room left open so the hall light shines in. Fear of small animals also can go on for several years, but usually goes away by the age of five.

At ages five, six, and seven, kids start showing fears about experiencing some type of bodily harm or injury. Chad, who is seven, is afraid that burglars are going to break in at night, even though (as his parents have pointed out) their house has an alarm system and is in a very safe neighborhood. Five-year-old Sage has begun expressing concerns about "getting hurt" or getting into an accident. Crystal, who has just turned six, told her dad, "I'm worried I'm going to be kidnapped!"

The early school years also are the time when fears of monsters and supernatural beings—ghosts, witches, mummies, werewolves, and vampires—occur (you'll probably find yourself being asked to check your child's closet and under the bed to make sure your son or daughter's room is "ghoul proof"). These fears often

Ages When Common Childhood Fears Begin

Age of child	Fears
Less than two years	Separation anxiety; stranger anxiety; fear of novel stimuli (loud noises, looming objects); fear of high places
Two to three years	Fear of the dark; fear of small animals
Five years	"Bad" or "mean" people; fear of bodily harm
Six years	Supernatural beings; sleeping alone; thunder and lightning
Seven to eight years	Fears based on media events
Nine years	School performance; physical appearance; fear of death

start with movies your child has seen. For example, Tara, age five, became fearful of witches after seeing the classic children's movie *The Wizard of Oz* for the first time. Seven-year-old Chen also became scared of witches after seeing the new Harry Potter film.

During kindergarten or first grade (at age five or six) kids become frightened of certain adults, whom they label "bad" or "mean." This can continue for several years or even for the rest of elementary school.

Your child may determine that someone is "bad" based on physical appearance—usually a physical appearance that's different from what he or she is used to. For instance, Rachel, a first grader, told her mom that she was scared of the homeless woman with the shopping cart—"the bad woman"—who was sitting on the front steps of the library. Tory, age five, was frightened of the man at the convenience store ("the bad man") whose arms were covered with tattoos.

The use of the word *mean* can be a child's way of describing adults in authority positions who are perceived as critical or strict, and who make the child feel anxious. These can be people who raise the volume of their voice a lot ("yellers"), or naturally have a loud voice, or use a particular tone of voice that is uncomfortable for your child.

Fear of thunder and lightning usually appears around the age of six and then continues for a year or two. During thunderstorms, six-year-old Simon sticks his fingers in his ears to try to block out the sound. In some cases fear of thunder and lightning goes on for a longer period of time, even through the fourth or fifth grade (age nine or ten). Beth, like Simon, first became frightened of thunder and lightning when she was six. She continued to have difficulty sleeping during thunderstorms until she was ten.

Also at age six, your son or daughter may begin to show anxiety about sleeping alone in his or her own bedroom. Your child may repeatedly ask to sleep in your bed or may "slip" into your bedroom (and your bed) during the middle of the night.

Kids also may be fearful at this age about being alone in places or situations where their moms or dads are not visible, even though they are readily accessible. For instance, your child may be uncomfortable being alone in a room of your home if you are in a different room. This was Keith's situation—he was unable to be alone in his playroom, even though his parents were right down the hall.

Your child also may be afraid of "minor separations" outside the home. This was the case for Kathryn, who insisted on being inside the stall of a public bathroom that her mother was using, rather than waiting just outside the stall door. Fears of sleeping alone and being alone should subside by the time your child is eight.

Fears begin to be influenced by media events—usually things your child sees on television (particularly the news)—at age seven or eight. The following fears frequently begin in this way:

- Fear of flying (following publicity surrounding the crash of an airplane)
- Fear of natural disasters such as hurricanes, tornadoes, floods
- Fear of manmade disasters—war, terrorist attacks, nuclear explosions, etc.
- Fear of diseases like AIDS and cancer
- Fear of being kidnapped

At around nine or ten, in the fourth or fifth grade, your child's fears turn to performance and social concerns. Fears of taking tests, giving oral reports, and performing in school in general come to the forefront. Your child also may begin expressing concerns about performance or "competence" in other things—like sports, playing an instrument, dance class, or any other nonacademic or out-of-school activity. At this age kids also become concerned with their physical appearance and others' (particularly peers') perceptions of them and whether they are "popular" and have enough friends.

This too is the time when your child may become preoccupied with the concept of his or her own—and others'—mortality and fearful of death. Shortly after her dog died, nine-year-old Sharon started to worry about what would happen *to her* when she died. Margaret, a fifth grader, began worrying about her parents dying after her grandfather passed away.

All these fears—about performance, social status, and death—can continue until your child is eleven or twelve years old. Some even may persist (with changes appropriate to your child's increasing age and changing developmental stage) into adolescence.

I Fears Are Universal

:h has shown there is consistency among childhood fears. As
oned earlier, kids with completely different backgrounds—
different nationalities, religions, financial circumstances, etc.—are
facing the same types of fears and at the same ages. One way this
can be understood is by considering the adaptive and protective nature of fear, especially in terms of its evolutionary significance.

For over a century, ethnologists—people who study survival patterns in the animal world—have known about the positive impact
that fear can have. In more recent years, psychologists also have
used this concept to help explain the development of fears and phobias in humans.

According to this evolutionary theory, people are "preprogram-
med" from birth to develop certain fears, ones that have, histori-
cally, contributed to the survival of our species. Through the process of natural selection children who possessed certain fears—and
avoided these objects and situations—were more likely to survive,
become adults, and reproduce. In this way, it is argued, fears have
become inbred into human beings, or, at the very least, the predis-
position or "preparedness" to develop these fears has been passed
down genetically, through the generations.

The evolutionary view helps explain why certain childhood
fears—such as separation anxiety, stranger anxiety, fear of heights,
fear of the dark, etc.—are so common among kids. In addition, it ex-
plains why the common childhood fears occur at certain times—
that is, when they are most advantageous to children's survival.
The "flip side" to this is that there are times when fears have
passed their normal developmental periods, when they no longer
are beneficial to your child, and actually become an impediment.

A good example of this is children's fears of heights. Your young
child's fear of high places can increase the likelihood of survival
(avoiding potentially damaging, or even lethal, falls). However, as
your child's motor coordination and visual acuity become more advanced this fear no longer may be adaptive. In fact, it actually may
hinder your child from showing a healthy sense of adventure and
becoming an autonomous and independent human being.

This is an example of how a normal childhood fear can persist too long and go "beyond normal," a subject I'll be discussing in more depth later on.

Environmental Influences on Normal Fears

Although the normal fears of childhood generally cross all "dividing lines" (ethnicity, religion, gender, etc.), some may be less likely to occur because of children's backgrounds and other environmental factors. For example, children who have grown up with a family pet (a dog, a cat) may be less likely to have a fear of small animals (or may have it to a lesser degree) than kids who haven't had this type of exposure. On the other hand, exposure to certain circumstances can make a child *more* fearful. For instance, research has shown that a fear of burglars is more prevalent among children raised in an urban, as opposed to a rural, environment.

> Although the normal fears of childhood essentially are universal, their presence can be influenced by environmental factors.

As I mentioned earlier, the events within our society, especially those that receive extensive media coverage, also can influence childhood fears. For example, while a fear of kidnapping—in both children and parents—certainly is not new, it seems to have grown in prevalence and intensity in recent years, probably because of the enormous media attention now given to child abductions.

What Is the Difference between "Fear" and "Anxiety"?

You've probably noticed that I've used both the words *fear* and *anxiety* in this chapter. Outside the mental health profession, especially among parents, "fear" often is thought to be less severe—more normal—than "anxiety." However, this really is not accurate. Fear can reach such high levels that it greatly, adversely affects your child's functioning. (In this case, the fear usually is termed a "phobia." We'll talk about this in the next chapter, where the focus is on childhood anxiety disorders.)

So what's the real difference between fear and anxiety? Although this is a straightforward enough question, there is no simple or single answer. The exact meaning of the two terms, and the differences between them, is debated even in psychiatric and psychological circles, and, thus, there is no consensus opinion on the matter.

Some professionals distinguish between fear and anxiety by the presence or absence of an object or situation—"fear" being associated with an outside "stimulus" (for example, fear of dogs, fear of public speaking, fear of flying, etc.; in other words, fear *of something*) and "anxiety," by contrast, being free-floating and not attached to a specific object or situation.

Although this point of view was popular for many years, current knowledge has led us to a different perspective today. Now experts believe that anxiety is a more global, or broader, phenomenon than fear. "Fear" is one type, or one form, of "anxiety." However, anxiety includes many more things than just fear. It also affects many aspects of your child's being, including feelings, behavior, and thoughts.

> **"Fear" is one type, or one form, of "anxiety." However, anxiety includes many more things than just fear.**

Anxiety includes generally uncomfortable feelings, such as being tense, nervous, "on edge," jittery, "uptight," jumpy, panicky, or, as we already discussed, fearful, which your child may describe using these words or in other ways. Nathan, age seven, told his mom, "My insides feel like they're jumping around!" Five-year-old Selena says she feels like she has "ants in her pants."

Anxiety also can appear as specific physical symptoms—like a racing heart or heart palpitations, tremulousness, dizziness, or "trouble breathing" (usually caused by hyperventilating). Brad, a fifth grader, told his dad, "My heart's pounding so hard it feels like it's going to come out of my chest!" (You might be interested to know that research consistently has shown that increased heart rate is the single most reliable indicator of anxiety.)

The physical symptoms produced by anxiety sometime like a medical problem. The most common of these are ~~l~~ and, especially, stomachaches. Your son or daughter may complain of stomach pain or queasiness, nausea, or feeling like he or she is going to vomit. Maria, a fourth-grade student, feels like she is going to throw up before taking tests. At gymnastic meets, six-year-old Tara always complains of "butterflies" in her stomach.

> **Anxiety affects:**
> • **Feelings**
> • **Behaviors**
> • **Thoughts**

Anxiety also includes nervous habits, like nail biting, hair pulling or twirling, a "restless leg," or knuckle cracking. Ten-year-old Katrina constantly redoes her ponytail, taking the elastic band out and then putting it in again. Tina is a hair "flipper," repeatedly jerking her head sideways to push the hair off her face.

Your anxious child may exhibit perfectionistic behavior. This was the case for Justine. At a parents' conference her kindergarten teacher said, "Justine is never happy with her drawings—she keeps erasing and doing them over, or else she throws them out and starts again."

Sometimes there are repetitious behaviors or rituals, where your child feels compelled to do something over and over again even though it really doesn't make sense. For instance, Brittany, age seven, has to have her dolls arranged in a very special way on her bed. Mathew, age ten, turns the light switches on and off three times whenever he enters or leaves a room.

"Not doing" certain things—avoiding or escaping contact with objects or situations—also is a type of anxious behavior. Sheila, who is afraid of dogs, wants to cross to the other side of the street when she sees a dog coming her way. Sometimes anxious behaviors are less obvious than this. For example, Janic   student never raises her hand when the teacher year-old Melissa goes to her friend's par

Ten-year-old Charlie had trouble "adjus at sleep-away camp. When Angela's fami schools, she'd call her mom from school allowed to come home. Being uncomfor situations—as in Charlie's and Angela's anxiety.

In addition to feelings and behaviors, anxiety includes certain types of thoughts, mental images, and ways of looking at or thinking about things. Your child may have worries, upsetting or catastrophic thoughts, or obsessions (including, possibly, "obsessional self-doubt," where your child repeatedly asks you for reassurance about something). Susie told her mom, "I get thoughts that something bad is going to happen to you." When riding in the car with his family, Malcolm almost always worries they'll get lost. Having upsetting dreams or nightmares is another way your child can show anxiety.

Because *anxiety* is a more comprehensive term than *fear*, it is the word I prefer to use when talking about the children who are the subject of this book (significantly, it also is the term experts use to describe the conditions that children with diagnosable anxiety experience—that is, "*anxiety* disorders," as opposed to "*fear* disorders"). However, there will be times when I use the two terms interchangeably, just to avoid the repetitiveness of using the word *anxiety* over and over again.

The Normal Anxieties of Children

Although hundreds, if not thousands, of research studies have investigated the fears that are normal during childhood, surprisingly few have looked at other forms of anxiety. What little research has been done on this, however, suggests there are certain, specific anxiety symptoms—apart from fears—that also are experienced during a child's normal development. In other words, children can have certain kinds of anxiety symptoms—besides fears—and still be normal too.

Our research group conducted two studies that addressed this subject. I'm highlighting them here not because of my own personal involvement with them, but because they are the only two investigations in this area—to my knowledge—where the "normalness" of the children clearly was established. To participate in our studies, the children had to have no history of any type of psychiatric disorder (this was determined from extensive interviews of the kids and their parents) and they could not have had any contact with a mental health professional. (Studies conducted by other researchers in this area have not taken these measures to ensure their children were normal. They have included kids from entire school classrooms or entire schools, who may or may not have had psychiatric or psychological problems.)

In our first study, reported in the *Journal of Clinical Child Psychology* in 1997, we looked at worrying—an anxiety symptom prevalent in children with anxiety *disorders* (anxiety conditions that warrant a psychiatric diagnosis)—in fifty-five normal children using a questionnaire. We found that around one-quarter of the children had "intense worries," that is, worries that are frequent and disturbing, most of which were related to *schoolwork* and *separation anxiety* concerns ("that my parents might abandon me"; "that my parents might die"; "getting lost," and the like).

In another, more comprehensive study, we looked at ninety different anxiety symptoms—not just worries—in sixty-two normal children, based on the children's and their parents' responses to interview questions. Again, as in our study on worrying, we found that some of the normal children had anxiety symptoms. The sidebar on the following page lists the anxiety symptoms, including fears, that were reported most frequently.

Children can have anxiety symptoms and still be normal.

An interesting postscript to the study I just described was that during the four years following the study, repeated reevaluations of the children showed that *virtually none* of them—including the ones who had anxiety symptoms—developed an anxiety disorder.

What do all of these research findings mean to you as a parent of a possibly anxious child? Just like the common fears of childhood, your child may experience other manifestations of anxiety (certain worries, anxious behaviors, etc.) as part of his or her normal development. And the presence of these normal anxiety symptoms may not have any significance later. As you've just seen, c^ild
have these symptoms may remain free from an anxiety anxiety disorder, as they get older.

Anxiety Symptoms in Normal Children

Anxiety symptom	Frequency (%)
Overly concerned about competence	35%
Excessive need for reassurance	31%
Fear of heights	23%
Fear of public speaking	22%
Somatic (physical) complaints	19%
Anxious avoidance of contact with others	19%
Fear of the dark	19%
Excessive worry about past behavior	18%
Self-consciousness	18%
Fear of harm befalling attachment figure	18%
Excessive worry about the future	15%
Fear of dressing in front of others	15%

Is "Normal" Different for Boys and Girls?

Most people assume that girls, normally, are more fearful or anxious than boys. Research, though, has not always supported this assumption. Although girls may be more apt to readily express these types of feelings (boys often learn to keep quiet and put on a "tough front" when they are frightened), studies that have looked at this issue show the two sexes really are more alike than you might think.

People assume that girls are more fearful or anxious than boys. The research literature on this, however, is far from conclusive.

For example, in the two studies I just described, there were no gender differences for fears, worries, or any of the other anxiety symptoms:

- In our questionnaire study of worries, boys and girls had the same total number of worries, the same number of "intense" worries, and the same content to their worries.
- In our interview study, there were no differences between boys and girls in the frequency of common anxiety symptoms (see the sidebar on the facing page), including fears.

Why is this important to you? Because as parents you may be using different standards to judge your sons and daughters—standards that, as we have just seen, aren't necessarily supported by fact.

So How Much Anxiety Is Too Much?

Since kids have fears and other anxiety symptoms as part of their normal development, how do you know when your child's anxiety is no longer normal—that it's "crossed the line" or gone "beyond normal"?

A good place to start is by completing the Child Anxiety Checklist on page 17. If your child has two parents, it would be helpful for your child's other parent, too, to answer the questions independently, since both of you may not have the same exact perception of your child. (Kids don't just look different to their parents. As you know, they often actually behave differently in front of their moms and dads.) An extra copy of the checklist is available at the back of the book for this purpose.

The checklist includes fifteen anxiety symptoms that frequently are present in kids who have anxiety problems. By completing the questionnaire and analyzing the results you'll begin to get a picture of your child's anxiety profile. I say "begin to get a picture" because the presence of any—or many—of these symptoms does not by itself mean your child has an anxiety problem. We need to get more information about each symptom before we know whether a problem exists. To be specific, we need to establish whether any of the anxiety symptoms that are present are *clinically significant*.

Anxiety symptoms are clinically significant because they either:

- Cause your child or your family considerable *distress* or
- Interfere with your child's *ability to function* in some aspect of life.

When symptoms disrupt functioning, they interfere with your child's ability to engage in age-appropriate activities and meet age-expected norms, like forming and maintaining friendships and meeting expectations at school (going to school regularly, completing homework on time and in an acceptable form, ability to take tests and give oral reports in front of the class, etc.).

Clinically significant anxiety symptoms are severe enough that they warrant attention and, most probably, intervention. In simpler terms, "clinically significant" is just another way of saying that your child's anxiety symptom is a problem.

Patty's mother and father completed the Child Anxiety Checklist about their eight-year-old daughter. They agreed that Patty has two of the items on the list—"trouble making friends because of excessive shyness" and "anxiety when in social situations." However, despite the fact that Patty's shyness causes some difficulties in making new friends, she does have two close friends her own age. Also, although Patty is somewhat uncomfortable at birthday parties and other social gatherings of kids her age, she goes to these activities without protest.

Patty's parents checked "yes" for two of the anxiety symptoms on the checklist. Although Patty clearly has anxiety symptoms, are they clinically significant? Does she have an anxiety problem?

To determine this, Patty's parents rated her anxiety symptoms using the form on page 18. You should do the same for each of the items you said "yes" to on the checklist, recording your ratings on that form. An extra copy of it is at the back of the book if your child's other parent is going to fill it out too.

1. *Rate the degree of distress each anxiety symptom causes your child and/or your family.* Using a 3-point scale, rate each anxiety symptom for the level of distress it causes. Use a "1" to

The Child Anxiety Checklist

Does your child . . .	Yes	No
Have recurrent stomachaches or headaches, for which there is no medical cause?	☐	☐
Have fears that are excessive (more intense than those of other children of similar age) or inappropriate for his or her age?	☐	☐
Have "nervous habits," such as nail biting, "restless legs," knuckle cracking, playing with hair, etc.?	☐	☐
Worry a lot? About a lot of different things?	☐	☐
Complain of upsetting thoughts or pictures (mental images)?	☐	☐
Engage in repetitive behaviors that must be performed but don't "make sense"?	☐	☐
Appear overly concerned or perfectionistic about performance in certain activities, either in or outside of school?	☐	☐
Exhibit anxiety when in social situations or when he or she is the center of attention?	☐	☐
Have trouble making friends because of excessive shyness?	☐	☐
Have frequent nightmares or bad dreams?	☐	☐
Tend to avoid or run away from frightening, but not dangerous, things (as opposed to confronting the feared object or situation)?	☐	☐
Get nervous in new situations or unfamiliar places?	☐	☐
Have a history of experiencing or witnessing a traumatic event, one that threatened his or her own, or someone else's, physical well-being?	☐	☐
Need a lot of reassurance?	☐	☐
Have trouble with changes in routine or a change in plans?	☐	☐

Child Anxiety Checklist Ratings

Checklist item (describe)	Ratings ("1," "2," or "3")	
	Distress	Functioning
_____	_____	_____
_____	_____	_____
_____	_____	_____
_____	_____	_____
_____	_____	_____
_____	_____	_____
_____	_____	_____
_____	_____	_____

indicate the anxiety symptom does not cause your child and/ or your family distress, a "2" to indicate the anxiety symptom causes your child and/or your family some distress, or a "3" to indicate the anxiety symptom causes your child and/or your family a lot of distress.

2. *Rate the extent to which each anxiety symptom interferes with your child's functioning.* Again using a 3-point scale, go back to each anxiety symptom you checked and rate it: "1" if it does not interfere with your child's functioning, "2" if it interferes to some extent with your child's functioning, or "3" if it interferes a lot with your child's functioning.

Clinically Significant Anxiety Symptoms

Any item that you rated a "3"—either for "distress" or for "interference with functioning" (or both)—is present at a clinically significant level. This means that your child's anxiety, at least in this particular area, is beyond normal—it is an anxiety problem.

Timmy is a six-year-old who is obsessed with making sure his toy cars are lined up "just right." He spends several hours a day doing this and, as a result, is late getting places, including school. His parents have been unsuccessful at changing his behavior. When they try to pull him away from his cars, Timmy gets "hysterical" and even, at time, threatens them.

Timmy's parents rated him as having clinically significant anxiety. They gave him a "3" for distress and a "3" for interference with functioning. (Just to let you know, Timmy also has several other anxiety symptoms that are clinically significant too.)

Eight-year-old Gail is a "worry wart." She worries about so many things that it's hard for her parents to keep track. She worries about how well she does at different things—gymnastics, band, and soccer. She also worries about bad things happening—like getting into a car accident, getting sick, or something awful happening to her parents. Gail also spends a lot of time worrying about what other kids think of her.

Gail's parents rated her worrying as causing her a lot of distress—a "3"—but gave it only a "2" for its effect on her functioning.

Nevertheless, with the one "3" Gail's worrying clearly is an anxiety problem.

Subclinical Anxiety Symptoms

Anxiety items that receive at least one "2" rating—and no "3"s—are considered to be at a *subclinical* level. Subclinical symptoms can be more difficult to interpret than clinically significant ones. They're not of sufficient severity to be considered "an anxiety problem," but they still do impact your child's and your family's life.

Remember Patty, the girl with the social anxiety symptoms? Patty falls into this subclinical category. Although she is shy and somewhat uncomfortable in social situations, Patty has close friends and participates in social activities with her peers. Her anxiety symptoms do not greatly affect her functioning, nor do they cause her a lot of discomfort. Her parents gave her "2"s for both of her symptoms.

Tamika, a perfectionistic fourth grader, also received subclinical ratings from her parents. Tamika's perfectionism shows itself mostly when she's doing her homework. She's so concerned about how good a job she's doing that she keeps checking her work. Consequently, it takes her more time to finish her homework (about thirty extra minutes) than it should. This means she has less after-school time to be with her friends.

Although her perfectionism causes her some distress, Tamika's parents do not feel it's severe enough to warrant a "3." The same is true of its impact on her functioning—they don't think any aspect of her life is impaired to a great extent.

Dina, a third grader, becomes anxious when there are changes in her plans or routine. For example, she gets uncomfortable if the teacher changes the order of things, like having reading class before spelling (spelling *always* comes first), or if recess has to be held inside because of the weather instead of outside on the playground, as is usual.

Dina's parents' ratings indicate their daughter has a subclinical level of anxiety. Although they do not see her anxiety as greatly affecting her functioning, it does cause her some distress—easily warranting a "2."

It's a good idea for you to keep track of your child's subclinical anxiety symptoms. While they are not a serious problem now, it is possible that they may progress, worsen, and become clinically significant later on. On the other hand, they may lessen—or go away completely—as your child gets older, without your necessarily having "to do something" about them. Unfortunately, there is no way to know for sure which outcome is likely for your child.

However, you can get some sense of the meaningfulness, and possible outcome, of your child's subclinical anxiety symptoms by looking at them a bit more closely. Are they different from the ones I mentioned earlier, when discussing the normal anxieties of children? (For example, if your child is a worrier, are the worries about schoolwork and separation issues—the worries that research showed often were present in normal kids—or is your child worried about other types of things, things not typical of normal children?) Does your child have many subclinical anxiety symptoms, or just one or two? For those anxiety symptoms your child has, were there subclinical ratings for *both* distress and impairment, or just one or the other?

Children with subclinical anxiety symptoms (and no clinically significant ones) often are described as anxious, but do not meet criteria for an anxiety disorder. Because they are not diagnosable, their situation may be overlooked or minimized, even though these kids and their families may benefit from some help.

Even if your child only has subclinical anxiety symptoms, you will get a tremendous amount out of this book. Each of the chapters in Part II contains a section with practical things you can do to help your child decrease his or her anxiety. In addition to helping your child feel better now, taking action at this time may increase the likelihood that your child's anxiety symptoms will not worsen and become an anxiety disorder later on.

Nonsignificant Anxiety Symptoms

You may have checked some items on the Child Anxiety Checklist that do not cause your child or your family distress or interfere with your child's functioning. Rated as "1"s, they're not subclinical or clinically significant.

However, if you took the time to pick up this book, it's unlikely that all of your child's anxiety symptoms will fall into this category. If they do, then maybe what you initially were concerned about really shouldn't be a concern after all.

This was the situation with five-year-old Mary. Knowing that anxiety problems run in their family (Mom, herself, has been diagnosed with an anxiety disorder), Mary's parents have been "on alert" for the possibility that their child might have similar problems. They observed that Mary has several nervous habits—like biting her nails and playing with her hair. She also is somewhat fearful of dogs, thunderstorms, and "monsters."

After reading this chapter, Mary's parents realize that their child's fears (of dogs, thunderstorms, and "monsters") are normal for her age. Also, they rated her nervous habits as a "1"— "nonsignificant"—for both distress and interference with functioning.

Mary's parents are now happy to know that despite their initial concern their daughter does not have an anxiety problem. In fact, based on the checklist results, it would be hard to make a case that she's overly anxious at all.

When Normal Fears Go beyond Normal

Using "distress" and "interference with functioning" to determine whether an anxiety symptom is "a problem" works for virtually all of the anxiety symptoms your child may experience, with one exception. The normal fears of childhood that we talked about earlier often cause children a lot of distress and interfere with their functioning, yet still are considered normal. But for some kids these fears go from normal to abnormal. So how do you know this has occurred? By looking at the age-appropriateness and intensity of the fears.

Normal fears can become abnormal if they are age-inappropriate or excessive.

In fact, the second item on the Child Anxiety Checklist asks whether your child has fears that are age-inappropriate or excessive—the two criteria that experts in this field use to establish when childhood fears have progressed beyond normal. If a child's fear is either age-inappropriate or excessive, it's considered an anxiety problem.

Age-Inappropriate Fears

When your child's fears appear in the "wrong" developmental period, or linger and persist past their expected lifespan, they are age-inappropriate.

As an example, let's look at the common childhood fear of strangers. This fear appears in almost all infants at some time between seven and twelve months and continues in some children up to the age of five. If your child has a fear of strangers after this, it's developmentally inappropriate and may be a problem area.

This was the case for Sandy, a seven-year-old who would crouch behind furniture whenever she met someone for the first time. Eight-year-old Frank also had this problem—but instead of hiding like Sandy, he'd become mute, wouldn't speak at all, in front of strangers.

How could these children's parents have known their kids' fears were developmentally inappropriate? First, they could use the information in this chapter on the normal age ranges of common childhood fears. They also might consult with professionals who are very familiar with children's typical behavior—like their kids' pediatricians or teachers—or they could talk to other parents about their children to get some idea of what they've been through. Obviously, the more information you obtain, the better position you'll be in to see where your child's behavior fits in.

Eight-year-old Benjamin is experiencing age-inappropriate separation anxiety. A lot of days he's afraid to leave his mom to go to school. Taylor, age nine, doesn't have trouble going to school, but she won't sleep alone in her own room—she keeps slipping into her parents' bed in the middle of the night.

Both of these kids are too old to be experiencing normal separation anxiety. The first signs of separation anxiety—such as infants' crying when they are separated from their mothers—usually appear by the age of two. After that, the fear may show up again at different times (like when your child first enters preschool or kindergarten) until the age of five or six. If Benjamin's and Taylor's parents had this information, they would have known their children were past the normal period for this type of behavior. Then they could have taken action to help their kids get rid of their fears.

Jasmine's parents could have benefited from knowing more about kids' fears of the dark. Until the age of eight it's normal for children to need a nightlight in their bedroom and their door left open, so light from the hall shines in. But Jasmine is eleven and she *still* can't go to sleep without the nightlight and the door wide open. Given her age, her fear of the dark is developmentally inappropriate.

Excessive Fears

Even if a fear occurs at a time that's developmentally appropriate, the fear can be excessive if it's more intense than what's usually experienced by a child of that particular age.

Four-year-old Jennifer's fear of small animals is age-appropriate—it falls within the "right" developmental period (between the ages of two and five)—but it's not normal because it's excessive. Jennifer's so fearful of cats that she's afraid to leave the house because she might, by chance, run into one.

Judging a fear as excessive can be tricky—it's a matter of degree. In Jennifer's case it's pretty clear that her fear is excessive, but for other kids it's not always that clear. Remember Sheila, the girl who wanted to cross the street when she saw a dog coming her way? Unlike Jennifer, Sheila's fear is not excessive. Wanting to escape contact with an animal that's actually present is much less extreme than avoiding leaving the house when there's no animal in sight.

Ten-year-old Joshua, like Jennifer, has a fear that's age-appropriate but excessive. He's been scared of thunder and lightning since he was six, the age when this fear often first appears in kids. It's normal for kids to have this fear even up to the age of twelve, to have feelings of anxiety during thunderstorms, be somewhat fearful of going out of the house during storms, and, if the thunder and lightning are happening at bedtime, have some trouble sleeping.

But Joshua's behavior is much more extreme than this. He gets severe stomachaches during thunderstorms, often to the point of throwing up. If the storm is at night, he can't go to sleep even *after* the thunder and lightning are over. He's so concerned about the possibility there might be a thunderstorm that he keeps checking the weather forecast—even on sunny days. Finally, he absolutely will not leave his home—even during the daytime—if there's a thunderstorm.

From infancy until the age of five, many kids show signs of separation anxiety. Karen, who is five years old, is at the tail end of the normal developmental period for this fear, but her separation anxiety has gone too far to be considered normal. While many kids have trouble separating from their moms during the first few days or weeks of kindergarten, Karen's still having this problem at the middle of the school year.

If it's not clear to you whether your child's fear has crossed over the line from normal to excessive, you should seriously consider consulting a mental health professional who has experience in making these distinctions. While normal childhood fears usually are transient and go away on their own, excessive (or abnormal) fears generally require intervention or they will continue—sometimes even for life. Therefore, it really is in your and your child's best interest to find out now whether or not there is a problem.

Dealing with Normal Fears

The normal fears of childhood—even though normal—still cause children a lot of distress and can interfere with their functioning. (As I mentioned earlier, it's for this very reason that the traditional criteria of "distress" and "interference with functioning" aren't used to identify what's abnormal when it comes to fears.)

Normal childhood fears—that are age-appropriate and not excessive—usually aren't targeted by mental health practitioners for intervention, because they are developmentally appropriate (normal) and usually go away on their own. However, even though your child may not need professional help, there are many things that you, as a parent, can do to help your child get through these fears faster and with less discomfort and fewer adverse effects.

Much of the information contained in Part II of this book will be very useful to you with this. Even though these chapters have been written primarily with the parents of children with anxiety disorders in mind, the methods outlined for approaching and overcoming fears and anxiety will help you too to help your child.

By now you should have a pretty good idea of whether your son or daughter is an anxious child and whether the anxiety symptoms are causing a problem. In the next chapter I discuss the specific types of anxiety problems that occur in elementary-school-age children. Let's see whether your child fits any of these descriptions.

2 THE MANY FACES OF CHILDHOOD ANXIETY

Lily definitely has an anxiety problem. Her mom completed the Child Anxiety Checklist in Chapter 1 and found out that she has a number of anxiety symptoms, all of which are interfering with her school and home life.

Although Lily's mom now feels certain she has a problem, she doesn't really understand what the problem is. She knows about some of the childhood anxiety disorders—separation anxiety disorder, obsessive–compulsive disorder—from articles she's read in parents' magazines. But exactly what type of problem does Lily have?

By now you've completed the Child Anxiety Checklist as Lily's mother did. You, too, probably believe your child has an anxiety problem but are still unsure about what kind.

The different types of anxiety problems—the anxiety *disorders—*that children experience are described in the American Psychiatric Association's *Diagnostic and Statistical Manual of Mental Disorders.* The DSM, as it's commonly called, is the psychiatric classification or diagnostic system used in the United States and in much of the rest of the world. From time to time, as new knowledge about psychiatric disorders accumulates, the DSM goes through the process of revision, so a number of updated versions have been published.

Of all the anxiety disorders contained in the current version of the DSM, six are potentially relevant to you as the parent of an anxious child.

This chapter contains brief descriptions of the disorders (they're

Anxiety Disorders in Preadolescent Children

Separation anxiety disorder

Generalized anxiety disorder

Social anxiety disorder

Specific phobia

Obsessive–compulsive disorder

Posttraumatic stress disorder

discussed at length in Part II) so you can begin to see if any look like what your child is experiencing.

It's not always easy to know for sure which anxiety disorder, or disorders, your child has. Although the information included here should help you, I want to emphasize that the formal diagnosis of any psychiatric condition ultimately should rest in the hands of a qualified mental health professional.

Separation Anxiety Disorder

Children with separation anxiety disorder have a persistent fear of being separated from their mothers, fathers, or other people they are very attached to. If your child becomes overly anxious at the prospect of being apart from you, or someone else he or she is attached to, he or she may have this anxiety disorder.

As moms are most often the ones children's separation anxiety is directed toward, for the purpose of this chapter I will address you as if you are the parent of an anxious child and assume that the separation-related fears are connected to you. *Please understand this is just for the sake of convenience.* A child's fear of separation can be connected to any family member—a grandparent (especially one who lives in or very near your child's home), an older sibling—or even someone outside the family who is very important to your child.

If your son or daughter has separation anxiety disorder, it's very likely you are seeing avoidance behavior. These are ways your child tries to prevent separation from occurring. Your child may refuse or be extremely reluctant to be apart from you in many or just a few select situations. These situations can be ones that are extremely important to your child's continuing development, such as going to school, or less critical, such as going to sleep-away camp. They may involve being at home without you or away from home without you or both.

> A child with separation anxiety disorder may be afraid to leave home without you or be at home without you or have anxiety in both types of situations.

Eight-year-old Noriko has anxiety about being at home without her mother. She screams to her mom, "Don't leave me here with the babysitter!" Kevin, a second grader, grabs on to his mother's legs to try to keep her from going food shopping, even though his father and sister are going to stay home with him.

Eleven-year-old Amy doesn't have trouble being at home without her mom, but she does have anxiety doing certain things away from home. She's not able to go to sleepovers at her friends' homes—she feels sick to her stomach and has to be picked up early. She also refuses to go to sleep-away camp, even though most of her friends spend their summers at the same camp in New Hampshire.

Nine-year-old Noah's anxiety about leaving home is even more severe than Amy's. He refuses to go to school, becomes hysterical and threatens his mom, "I'll kill myself if you make me go." He also can't handle going to day camp in the summer. Alexis, a first grader with separation anxiety, is unable to go next door to play with her friend—she "feels sick" and has to go home. To have a play date her friend has to come over to Alexis's house.

Does your child act very "clingy" with you or demand excessive physical contact? Kids with separation anxiety often behave this way. For example, nine-year-old Kate always wants to sit in her mother's lap while the family watches TV. Marilyn, a fifth grader, "bear hugs" her mom so hard that she feels like she's being crushed.

At home, eight-year-old Tommy follows his mother from room to room. Youngsters with separation anxiety often "shadow" their moms like this (which, understandably, can be very annoying to parents). In addition, children with separation anxiety may be uncomfortable being alone in their own rooms, even in the daytime.

Your child may have trouble sleeping alone at night. Nine-year-old Ellen repeatedly asks her mother, "Can I *please* sleep in your bed tonight?" Seven-year-old Jose doesn't ask his parents if he can sleep with them—he just slips into their bed in the middle of the night. When Dad insists he return to his own room, Jose cries, screams, and begs to be allowed to stay.

As you can see, children with separation anxiety show their anxious feelings in different ways. When anticipating separation, your child may shake, cry, scream, hyperventilate, complain of a stomachache (or of "feeling sick"), "panic," cling to you, throw a tantrum, or make threats about self-harm (as was the case for Noah). During separations your son or daughter may seem "depressed" and withdrawn or nervous and "hyped up."

Do you receive numerous telephone calls from your child when the two of you are apart? Children with separation anxiety often do this because it makes them feel closer to their parents during separations, or it's an attempt to convince their folks to come home or come and get them (if the child is away from home). For example, when left at home with a babysitter on Saturday night, Cassandra, age eleven, keeps calling her mom's cell phone—*every fifteen minutes*—asking when she and her dad will be coming home.

A child with separation anxiety also may have upsetting thoughts, worries, and/or nightmares that focus on separation-related themes. Kids may worry (or have bad dreams) that something awful will happen to them—that they'll be kidnapped or killed and never see their parents again. Instead, or in addition, your child may have distressing thoughts or dreams about something terrible happening to *you*—that you'll get sick or be in an accident and die (which would result in "permanent separation").

Michael's mom picks him up every day after school. But if she is even five minutes late (which happens occasionally because of traffic), he worries that she's been in a car accident. By the time she gets to the school Michael is sitting on the curb crying. He's convinced she's been killed and he'll never see her again.

Generalized Anxiety Disorder

Children with generalized anxiety disorder are, first and foremost, worriers. They worry excessively about a lot of different things, and most of their worries are about the possibility of something terrible or "catastrophic" happening.

If your child has this anxiety disorder, you probably frequently hear "But Mom [or Dad], *what if* _____?" Kids like this often are described as "worry warts" or "nervous nellies."

Ten-year-old Marcia always seems to be worried that something terrible is going to happen. During thunderstorms she worries that lightning will strike her house. When riding in the car with Mom or Dad she worries they might get lost or be in an accident. Before starting a new school year she's overly anxious about what her new teacher will be like. Marcia also has concerns that are not typical for a child her age. For example, she worries about her family's finances. She's also anxious about things that aren't going to happen until she is much older, like whether she'll get into a good college.

> **Children with generalized anxiety disorder often are described as "worry warts" or "nervous nellies."**

Mathew, an extremely bright straight-A student, is always worried about his grades. He gets anxious before tests and worries afterward that he might not have done well. When report cards are due, he's so nervous he can't sleep. Like Mathew, your child may have worries that are unrealistic or irrational.

In addition to worries about school performance, your child may be overly concerned, or even "a perfectionist," about performance in nonacademic activities—like sports or playing a musical instrument. Kids like this often need a great deal of reassurance from their parents or others (their teachers, coaches, etc.) that they are "doing okay."

Although worrying about the future is most characteristic of generalized anxiety disorder, your child also may be overly concerned and preoccupied with situations that have already taken place.

Eleven-year-old Abigail repeatedly replays past events in her head, concerned about whether she did or said the "right" thing.

In addition to worrying, kids with generalized anxiety disorder experience physical manifestations of anxiety. Your child may have recurrent stomachaches, headaches, or other types of aches and pains. The physical symptoms, however, usually do not follow a clear-cut or obvious pattern (as opposed to separation anxiety disorder, where children experience physical problems only when anticipating or confronting separation situations). However, if you question your child about what he or she is thinking about, you may find that upsetting thoughts and worries trigger the physical problems.

Kids with generalized anxiety disorder show their anxiety in many other ways as well. Some have difficulty falling or staying asleep or problems with concentration. Your child may be generally "uptight," jittery, nervous, "on edge," "hyper," or irritable. You may notice nervous habits, such as nail biting, fidgeting, knuckle cracking, and playing with or "twirling" hair.

Although avoidance behavior usually is not obvious in children with generalized anxiety disorder, if you look closely at these children's behavior, or get information about how they act in different environments (for example, from their teachers), you'll probably find that they engage in subtle forms of avoidance. Terry, for example, is uncomfortable traveling in a car—she's afraid there's going to be an accident. She closes her eyes or looks away from the road to decrease her anxiety. Sam, who lives in South Florida, worries during hurricane season. He avoids the weather report on TV and the radio, leaving the room or switching the channel or station. (On the other hand, some children who have worries like Sam do the opposite—they become preoccupied with checking the weather forecast.) Mary Beth doesn't participate in sports because she's afraid she won't do well. When the teacher asks a question in class, Erica never raises her hand—she's worried she won't give the right answer.

All of these children have avoidance behaviors. It's just that they're not as obvious, and, consequently, easily identifiable as those present in some of the other childhood anxiety disorders.

Social Anxiety Disorder

The key feature of social anxiety disorder, or *social phobia* as it also is termed, is an extreme, persistent fear of a social or performance situation. If your child is very afraid of being embarrassed in front of other people in certain social or performance situations—and tries to avoid these situations (or endures them with dread)—he or she may have this anxiety disorder.

There are two forms of social phobia—the *circumscribed* type and the *generalized* type. In the circumscribed form, your child is fearful of one or more specific situations. Some common circumscribed social phobias in children are:

- Public speaking (in front of the class)
- Eating/drinking in front of other people
- Undressing in front of others
- Urinating or defecating in public restrooms
- Blushing
- Performing in front of others (for example, in some type of recital, play, or sports event)

Nine-year-old Liam is terrified of giving book reports in front of the class. The night before, he gets extremely nervous. The morning he's scheduled to give the report, he tells his mother, "I'm sick. I can't go to school." Marcus, a fourth grader, can't eat in the school cafeteria with the other kids. He feels like everyone is watching him and is afraid he'll embarrass himself in some way. Seven-year-old Beth can't change into her gym clothes in the girls' locker room. She has to go into a bathroom stall so no one will see her. Jim, in the first grade, won't use the bathroom at school. He makes his mom pick him up at lunchtime so he can use the one at home.

Social phobias can seem like they're directed at school in general, but usually it's a specific situation at school that's causing the problem, like one of the ones I just mentioned. It also can be that your child is being teased or bullied by classmates.

For example, Frank, an overweight eight-year-old, desperately tries to get his mother to let him stay home from school. When Frank's mom went to the school to talk with his teacher about the problem, she discovered he was being teased about his size by some of the other boys in the class.

Is your child extremely anxious in almost all social situations? Then your son or daughter may have the generalized, rather than the circumscribed, form of social anxiety disorder. Kids with generalized social phobia usually are very uncomfortable with other kids, particularly those their own age. (They also can be anxious around adults, especially those they don't know well.) They frequently are very quiet or withdrawn at school and may have no or only one or two close friends or be able to form friendships only with younger kids.

Anna, a sixth-grade student, has generalized social phobia. Although she is three-quarters of the way through the school year, she's still uncomfortable with the other kids in her class. In fact she never talks to any of her classmates. If they talk to her, she responds with only one- or two-word answers. Although she has no friends at school, Anna does have a "best friend," Belinda, who lives in her neighborhood. But because Belinda is two grades behind her, Anna gets to see her only after school and on weekends.

Seven-year-old Charley, although a lot younger than Anna, also has generalized social phobia. He doesn't want to go to school, but his mother makes him go. At recess he stands off to the side by himself and doesn't play with any of the other kids. At lunchtime he eats in the cafeteria alone. Charley doesn't take part in any after-school activities. After school he does his homework and then entertains himself with TV or computer games.

Generalized social phobia is not shyness. Shyness does not cause the same level of distress or impact kids' functioning the way generalized social phobia does. If you have a shy child, he or she probably is able to do most of the things that "non-shy" children are able to do—it just may take your child a bit longer to become comfortable. (For this reason, shy children sometimes are described as "slow to warm up.") Kids with generalized social phobia, on the other hand, virtually never become comfortable in social situations—even with familiarity, they continue to be extremely anxious.

Children with social phobias—regardless of whether they have the circumscribed or generalized form of the disorder—have upsetting and catastrophic thoughts about being embarrassed in some way when anticipating or confronting their feared situations. For ex-

> **Generalized social phobia is not shyness.**
>
> **Shy children "warm up" over time, while children with generalized social phobia almost never do.**

ample, eleven-year-old Janice is afraid to talk to kids she doesn't know well because she's concerned she'll "look stupid." Andrew, a second grader, tells his mom he doesn't want to take part in show-and-tell because he's afraid he'll "mess up" and be embarrassed in front of the class. Imani, in third grade, won't raise her hand at school because she's afraid of "sounding dumb."

Children with social anxiety disorder try to avoid the social and performance situations that create anxiety, but if avoidance is not possible (usually because their parents won't allow it), they will endure the situations with a great deal of discomfort.

When anticipating or facing social or performance situations your child may have physical symptoms similar to those I've already described for the other types of anxiety disorders. In addition, children with social phobias can have trouble speaking, in different ways, when faced with their feared situations. Your child may not be able to speak at all or have limited speech (like Anna) or may have speech "irregularities" such as stuttering or a shakiness in the voice, awkward hesitations or lengthy delays when beginning to speak, nervous coughing or clearing of the throat that interrupt speech, or very rapid or slowed speech.

Children who are socially anxious can freeze up in other ways too, besides their speech. During her piano recital, ten-year-old Meagan completely "forgot" the piece she spent so much time practicing and memorizing. At her school soccer playoff, Tamara, the team's star player, just stood still—like she was immobilized—when the ball came her way.

Specific Phobia

Specific phobias are very much like social phobias—they are excessive and persistent fears—except that the fear is not about a social or performance situation. As with social phobias, children with specific phobias try very hard to avoid contact with the source of their fears, but when they have to confront them they always experience extreme anxiety.

Some specific phobias that are common in children are of:

- Dark places
- Small animals
- Insects
- Needles (injections; having blood drawn)
- Heights
- Swimming or being in or near deep water
- Flying
- Vomiting
- Enclosed places

You may notice that some of the items in this list are the same as ones included in the sidebar on normal fears in Chapter 1 (see page 5). That's because—as discussed in the last chapter—the normal fears that children experience growing up can persist beyond their expected developmental periods (becoming age-inappropriate) or, even if they are age-appropriate, they can be more severe than what's expected of children at that age. In these cases the normal fears of childhood have gone "beyond normal" and become phobias.

Although Jamie's fear of cats was "normal" when she was little, it went on and worsened when she got older. At ten she won't go to her best friend's house because her family has two cats. She also won't go into the pet store with her mom to buy dog food for their dog because she knows there are cats inside. Jamie even has trouble when she sees a cat in a movie or when there is a picture of one in a book or magazine.

Lindsey, a fifth grader, also has a fear that would be considered normal in a very young child but is a phobia because of her age. Because of her fear of heights she won't go on the balance beam in gym class, even though she knows she'll end up getting an F.

Fred has a different situation. At seven, his fear of the dark is age-appropriate, but it's so intense—so excessive—that it's a specific phobia. Fred's so terrified of the dark that he can't even stand in the doorway of his own room to turn on the light switch.

Children also can have specific phobias about other things that, although usually not classified as normal fears of childhood, frequently cause kids some degree of anxiety and discomfort. For phobic kids, though, the reactions are much greater than for normal kids.

For example, let's look at Hope, a second grader who is terrified of needles. Hope is so frightened of injections that she literally has to be forced to go to the doctor when she needs a shot or vaccination. First her parents have to physically restrain her to get her into the car. Then, when she's in the waiting room, they have to keep holding on to her or she'll run out of the building. While in the examining room, she screams nonstop even *before* she receives the injection.

As another example, consider nine-year-old Christian, who is panic-stricken about flying. For weeks before his family's vacation he's so nervous he has trouble falling asleep. He repeatedly tells his mom, "I don't want to go!" When it comes time to leave for the airport, he runs out of the house and keeps on going until his dad is able to catch up with him.

While no child likes to get sick and throw up, Carmen, a third-grade student, has a phobia about vomiting. She's consumed with the possibility of throwing up and avoids things she believes might cause her to vomit. She won't go on many of the rides at the amusement park (particularly the ones that involve spinning), even though she's never gotten sick on one before. She refuses to eat certain foods she thinks might make her throw up. She also becomes extremely anxious if she's been near someone who is sick or if she thinks she might be getting sick, because she's afraid an illness might cause her to vomit.

Nine-year-old Kevin is terrified of bees and wasps. Since he lives in the northern part of the United States, he has to deal with them only during the summer. But during these few months his life is severely restricted. He refuses to play outside with his friends or to go to day camp because of the outdoor activities.

Children often have specific physical signs of anxiety when anticipating encountering or actually encountering the source of their phobias. Every time Lauren saw a dog she told her dad, "My heart is beating really fast!" Whenever Chad's parents drove over a bridge (which was often since they lived in a coastal, metropolitan area), he said to his parents, "It feels like butterflies are jumping around in my tummy." Your child even may have panic attacks when facing his or her phobia.

If your child has a specific phobia, he or she also may have upsetting or catastrophic thoughts (which might be expressed out loud) about the feared object or situation. Evan, a fourth grader who is afraid of dogs, told his mom, "I'm afraid they'll bite me." Christian, who, as you'll recall, has a phobia about flying, said to his dad, "I'm frightened the airplane will crash!" Seven-year-old Cheyenne, who has a fear of small enclosed places, is afraid she'll get trapped in an elevator and that it will "run out of air."

Obsessive–Compulsive Disorder

Children who have obsessive–compulsive disorder either have obsessions—recurring and disturbing thoughts or images—or compulsions, repetitive behaviors performed in a "ritualized" manner, or both of these problems. Obsessions often cause kids a great deal of distress, while compulsions frequently are time-consuming and interfere with different aspects of day-to-day functioning.

Obsessions are different from the upsetting thoughts and worries that accompany many of the other childhood anxiety disorders. Obsessions are experienced as intrusive and "foreign" and as not making sense. They'll seem to your child as if they come "from nowhere" or "out of the blue" and from outside your child (it's for this reason that kids frequently have names for their obsessive–compulsive disorder, placing distance between it—the disorder—and themselves).

Also, obsessions are not about real-life problems or situations. The content of obsessions very often is violent, horrific, and abhorrent to your child or uncomfortably inappropriate in some other way.

Seven-year-old Shawna has an obsession. Several times a day she has a mental image of her house on fire and her parents being burned to death. She loves her parents and is horrified by the pictures that keep popping into her head. Bobbi, a fifth grader, has an obsession about being sexually molested by a family member. She knows that nothing like this has ever happened and feels tremendously guilty about having these thoughts.

Sometimes obsessions are just senseless, seemingly random thoughts that plague your child over and over again and cause him or her to feel "stuck." For example, Brian, a fourth grader, has obsessive thoughts about "the true meaning" of the word "death." Hallie, who is in second grade, keeps having the number "7" appear in her head. Eight-year-old Hiroko finds herself repeating, silently to herself, a list of things she likes to do.

Obsessive thoughts always are *resisted*. Your child will try very hard to ignore or suppress the obsession or may attempt to counter or "undo" it with another thought or series of thoughts. For example, Martha, a nine-year-old student at a private religious school, has blasphemous obsessive thoughts about God. She tries to "undo" the "bad" (sacrilegious) thoughts by immediately saying a special prayer—"good" thoughts—in her head.

Some children respond to their obsessions with ritualistic behaviors—compulsions—that you can see. For instance, Shawna, the girl I described a little earlier who has the fire obsession, reacts to her obsession by knocking three times on a table or another piece of furniture that is close by.

In Shawna's case the ritual she performs—the knocking—is not connected in any meaningful or realistic way to her obsession. While Shawna's logical self knows that her compulsion does not have the potential to undo or prevent the awful thing she imagines, she just can't stop herself from doing it. As for Shawna, your child's compulsions most probably do not accomplish what they're intended to achieve.

Even if you can see some connection between your child's obsession and compulsion, it will be obvious to you that the behavior is excessive or unreasonable. For example, Jennifer, an eight-year-old with an obsession about dirt and germs, washes all of her dolls by hand, with soap and water, every night. Ten-year-old Jeffrey, who has a similar obsession with dirt and germs, washes his hands twenty to thirty times a day.

While kids can have just obsessions or only compulsions, most children with obsessive–compulsive disorder have both of these problems. When compulsive behaviors occur in the absence of obsessions they usually are "arranging" or "ordering" rituals. Your child may feel compelled to (and spend a great deal of time) putting objects in certain positions relative to each other or performing certain activities in very specific sequences.

> While kids can have just obsessions or only compulsions, these problems most often occur together.

Eight-year-old Devon has to have her stuffed animals arranged in a very specific way. If they are not positioned "exactly right" she gets extremely upset and can't go to sleep. Eleven-year-old Nicole has a special order and manner for conducting her morning grooming activities, including brushing her teeth (from left to right—first the uppers, then the lowers, then repeat two more times) and showering (always beginning by washing her head and ending with her feet).

If your child has a compulsion, either in response to an obsession or just alone, he or she will become very upset if you try to prevent the activity. When Jacob's dad tries to stop him from doing his ritual (turning the light switch on and off multiple times), the child physically strikes out at him. Leslie, an eleven-year-old who repeatedly, compulsively checks and rechecks the locks on her bedroom windows, threatens her mother "I'll run away from home!" if she interferes with her daughter's ritual.

Posttraumatic Stress Disorder

Unlike the other anxiety disorders we've already discussed, to have this anxiety disorder children have to have been exposed to a traumatic event. By "exposed" I mean that your child either has directly expe-

> To have posttraumatic stress disorder, your child has to have been exposed—directly or indirectly—to a trauma.

rienced a trauma or else has observed someone else experiencing it.

The traumatic event must be a situation outside of your child's control. In other words, your child did not make it happen (as, for example, in the case of self-inflicted harm) and could not (within reason) have prevented it from happening.

Also, for the diagnosis of posttraumatic stress disorder, the trauma situation must include the threat of death or actual death, serious injury, or some other type of threat to the physical well-being of your child or others. Some examples of traumatic events that can result in children developing posttraumatic stress disorder include:

- A major car accident (particularly one involving fatalities or serious injuries)
- Physical abuse
- Sexual abuse
- Kidnapping
- Robbery (involving actual or threatened violence)
- War, terrorist attacks, and other "manmade" disasters
- Natural disasters (for example, floods, hurricanes, earthquakes, tornadoes), where there are actual or threatened losses of life

Children frequently react to experiencing or witnessing a trauma with fear or horror. If your child is young, however, he or she may react instead by becoming extremely agitated or appearing "out of it" or in "another world." This was the case for five-year-old Gabriela. For some time after the bomb scare at her school she looked like she was "in a daze."

After the trauma is over, children who develop posttraumatic stress disorder will keep reexperiencing the event in some way. After seeing her younger sister kidnapped from the playground, nine-year-old Brook had flashbacks of it in her head. Jay, a third grader who saw his friend struck by a car, keeps having distressing thoughts about what happened. Ten-year-old Ira has nightmares about the hurricane that destroyed his home. Emory, a kindergarten student molested in aftercare, re-creates what happened to her when she plays with her dolls.

Following the trauma your child may try to avoid things that are reminders of what happened. Your child may try to avoid or suppress thoughts or images of the trauma and/or refuse to talk about or be present during conversations about the traumatic event. Eric, a first grader, covers his ears and runs out of the room when he hears his parents discussing what happened to him.

Children with posttraumatic stress disorder often try to escape activities that involve being exposed to objects, situations, places, or people that remind them of the trauma. For instance, Shelly, described later, has not wanted to be in a car since the accident. After an unsuccessful kidnapping attempt, Paula can't look at men who resemble, in some way, the guy who tried to abduct her.

When your child must face things that are reminders of the trauma, he or she will become extremely anxious and upset. When they pass the intersection where the accident took place, six-year-old Sunee starts shaking and screams, "Mommy, watch out!!!"

Faye, who was placed in a foster home and then (fortunately) adopted by a very loving family, does not recall the physical abuse she suffered while living with her biological parents. Like Faye, children with posttraumatic stress disorder may seem to be suffering from some type of "amnesia," unable to remember the traumatic event or certain aspects of it.

Posttraumatic stress disorder often causes an increased level of general anxiety that can appear in several different ways. Kids may have difficulty falling or staying asleep or become very irritable or have frequent outbursts of anger. Your child may have difficulty concentrating (and, consequently, have school grades drop), or become hypervigilant and always "on guard." Some children develop an exaggerated startle response to loud noises or the sudden unexpected appearance of objects or people. Since the day of his trauma, Quinn's mom has noticed that he's very jumpy—he almost comes out of his seat whenever the telephone or doorbell rings.

Ever since the robbery, when she and her family were held up at gunpoint, Marta has seemed "detached" from other people—even her parents and her best friend. She's lost interest in many of her activities and is a lot less animated than she used to be. This kind of emotional detachment can occur in children with posttraumatic stress disorder.

Children also can lose the sense of "having a future" after being exposed to a trauma. Your child may no longer anticipate experiencing the positive events that normally take place growing older. For example, Whitney, age ten, can't picture entering middle school. Eleven-year-old Tess, who also has posttraumatic stress disorder, can't believe she'll ever get married and have children like her mom did. Miguel, an outstanding sixth-grade student who used to believe he eventually would go to a first-rate college, no longer sees himself going on with his education after high school.

Younger children with posttraumatic stress disorder sometimes show signs of regression following the trauma. It looks like they've lost developmental milestones that previously were obtained. After he and his family were robbed in their home, Craig, age six, began wetting his bed and speaking in "baby talk." After surviving a serious car accident, eight-year-old Shelly is sucking her thumb—a habit she outgrew two years ago—and having trouble separating from her mom.

Although posttraumatic stress disorder is one of the anxiety disorders that can appear in childhood, I will not be covering it in detail in Part II of this book, as I will the other anxiety disorders I've discussed in this chapter. That's because this particular anxiety disorder is not a problem, in my opinion, that should be handled by parents, even with the assistance of a self-help book.

If you think your son or daughter may have this anxiety disorder, please have your child evaluated by a qualified mental health professional, who can correctly diagnose and treat this problem for you.

What about "Panic Disorder"?

You may have noticed earlier that "panic disorder" was not included in the sidebar on page 28 that listed the anxiety disorders of childhood. That's because panic disorder very rarely occurs before adolescence. In fact, it usually begins in late adolescence or early adulthood.

Although panic *disorder* is extremely rare in elementary school-age children, panic *attacks* are not. Your child may have panic attacks as part of separation anxiety disorder, social anxiety disorder, a specific phobia, obsessive–compulsive disorder, or posttraumatic stress disorder.

If your preadolescent child is suspected of having panic disorder, in most cases he or she probably is suffering from separation anxiety disorder (the second most likely cause is a severe phobia). An expert in child anxiety disorders will be able to make this differential diagnosis accurately for you.

Can My Child Have More Than One Anxiety Disorder?

As you just read the descriptions of the specific anxiety disorders you may have found that your son or daughter seems to fit more than one of them. This is very common. In fact multiple anxiety disorders—where your child has two or more anxiety disorders at the same time—is the "rule" rather than the exception.

There are certain, specific anxiety disorders that tend to "go together." As one example, children with generalized anxiety disorder often also have phobias. In Part II, where each individual anxiety disorder is described at length, I'll tell you which anxiety disorders are most likely to co-occur. Also, as we'll discuss in Part II, once your child has had an anxiety disorder he or she may have a greater chance (than a child who has never had an anxiety disorder) of developing another (different) anxiety disorder in the future.

Is It Really an Anxiety Disorder, or Could It Be Something Else?

There are other psychiatric disorders that your child may have that can be mistaken, and misdiagnosed, as an anxiety disorder. On the other hand, your son or daughter may be given one of these other diagnoses, when, in actuality, he or she *really does* have an anxiety disorder.

The two nonanxiety disorders that are most likely to lead to this type of confusion are attention-deficit/hyperactivity disorder and depression. Since attention-deficit/hyperactivity disorder is more likely to occur in elementary-school-age children, let's start with it first.

Attention-Deficit/Hyperactivity Disorder

Attention-deficit/hyperactivity disorder, or ADHD as it is commonly known, and anxiety disorders share certain characteristics and, as a result, can be mistaken for each other. However, despite some overlap in symptoms there are a number of things that can help you distinguish between the two problems.

The main features of ADHD include (1) attention problems, (2) hyperactivity, and (3) impulsivity.

Attention Problems

Max's parents complain that their ten-year-old son doesn't listen. They have to keep repeating themselves because he doesn't respond. They don't know whether he really doesn't hear them—because of a hearing problem or some type of attention problem—or he's just choosing to ignore them. The parents of kids with ADHD often talk about their children in this way.

The attention problems of children with ADHD come from easy distractibility (by outside stimuli) and/or from daydreaming. Adam, a seven-year-old with ADHD, loses his concentration at school when he hears sounds—a siren or kids on the playground—or sees things moving outside the classroom window, like the branches of a tree swaying in the wind. Destiny, a fourth grader diagnosed with ADHD, is unable to keep track of what her teacher is saying because she's busy daydreaming about the trip her family is going to take this weekend to Disney World.

Children with anxiety disorders, like kids with ADHD, sometimes have difficulty paying attention and concentrating. However, when anxious children have attention problems it's because of upsetting or frightening thoughts or physical manifestations of anxiety (feeling jittery or "on edge"; stomachaches; headaches) that interfere with their ability to concentrate.

If your child has attention and concentration problems as part of an anxiety disorder, he or she probably—despite the problem—manages to do okay at school. On the other hand, if your son or daughter has ADHD, the teacher probably has said that your child has an "attention problem" (or a "behavior problem"; see below). This was the case for both Greg and Greta. Every quarter on his report card Greg's teacher comments that he has trouble paying attention in class. At the first parent–teacher conference of the year, Greta's teacher told her mom, "Greta often seems to be daydreaming and is having difficulty keeping up with the rest of the class."

Because the attention problems of kids with ADHD usually are pretty severe, they often have trouble with their grades even despite having average or above average abilities. Moreover, it's not uncommon for ADHD kids to have to repeat a grade level. By contrast it's *extremely* uncommon for an anxious child to have to do so.

Hyperactivity

Seven-year-old Donny has ADHD. His teacher complains that he's a disruptive influence in the classroom. Donny frequently leaves his seat without permission and pesters the other children around him, throwing spitballs and getting "physical" with them. He also has problems at home, like difficulty staying in his chair at the kitchen table throughout dinner. He doesn't seem to be able to play quietly by himself, frequently driving his mother crazy with his overly energetic behavior.

> **Children with ADHD are labeled by their teachers as having an "attention problem" or a "behavior problem."**

Kids with anxiety disorders can have certain behaviors—fidgeting, pacing, or nervous habits—that can be misinterpreted as "hyperactivity." True hyperactivity, though, as in Donny's case, has a more active or energetic quality to it and is more disruptive and inappropriate than the behaviors exhibited by children who have anxiety disorders.

Does your child seem to be in constant motion? Act somewhat inappropriately or "out of control"? Nine-year-old Claire, who is being treated for ADHD, initially behaved this way. She would move almost nonstop around her doctor's office—from one piece of furniture or object to the next.

Anxious children almost never behave like this. To the contrary, they usually are concerned—often to the point of being *overly* concerned—about behaving "correctly," being liked, and doing the "right thing." Unlike Claire, when Mathew, an eight-year-old with an anxiety disorder, first visited his therapist's office, he squirmed and fidgeted but never actually left his seat.

Impulsivity

Children with ADHD often do things "on impulse," without really thinking them through or considering the potential negative consequences of their actions.

Differences between Children with Anxiety Disorders and Children with ADHD

Anxiety disorder	ADHD
Teacher perceives child as well behaved.	Teacher perceives child as a behavior problem.
Child gets along with/is liked by peers.	Child often is ostracized or rejected by peers.
Child usually gets good grades.	Child often gets poor grades.
Child tends to keep things neat and well organized.	Child often misplaces or loses things.
Attention span not usually a major problem.	Attention span very often a major problem.
Thoughts can be upsetting/fearful.	Thoughts often take the form of pleasant daydreams.
Child may have a marked startle response, for example, to sudden loud noises, etc.	Child is distracted by, but not startled by, external objects and situations.
Child is well coordinated.	Child is clumsy.
Equally common among boys and girls.	More common among boys.

Does your child seem to act "without thinking" or not "plan ahead"? Does the teacher complain that your child blurts out answers to questions without first raising his or her hand? Or shoves other children out of the way to be first on line? Kids with ADHD often behave like this.

Sarah, a fifth-grade student with ADHD, gets into trouble at school because she frequently talks "out of turn," whispering to the girl next to her while her teacher is talking. Alejandro's mother is frightened that her son will get hurt doing one of his "daredevil" bicycle tricks.

Sometimes an anxious child can appear impulsive. David, a

seven-year-old with separation anxiety disorder, seems to act impulsively when faced with the possibility of being apart from his mom. When she tries to leave him home with a babysitter, he runs out of the house and after her car, oblivious to the other cars on the road.

"Escape behavior"—running away from something feared—like David's is very common in children who have anxiety disorders. You also may find that if your anxious child is in need of reassurance about some potentially anxiety-producing event, he or she may butt into an ongoing conversation. This too can make your child look impulsive.

Kids with ADHD are impulsive more consistently—more of the time and in many different types of situations—than anxious kids. In addition, their impulsive behaviors are not "fueled" by anxiety.

As a general rule, if your child's teacher has not repeatedly complained about your child's attention or behavior—if you have not received numerous telephone calls or notes from the school, and comments on report cards or during parent–teacher conferences—it's unlikely your child has ADHD.

The Co-occurrence of Anxiety and ADHD

Now that I've pointed out how children with anxiety disorders and ADHD differ, we need to consider that the two conditions can occur *simultaneously* in your child. This obviously complicates matters, making the job of determining which problem or problems your child is experiencing that much more difficult.

Interestingly, it's only relatively recently that the possible co-occurrence of anxiety disorders and ADHD was recognized. For many years it had been assumed that what were called "internalizing disorders," because they were experienced primarily "on the inside," such as anxiety and depression, could not coexist in children with the so-called "externalizing disorders"—those experienced primarily "on the outside," that is, through observable behavior—such as ADHD. In fact, because of this thinking many of my early research studies on children with anxiety disorders included ADHD kids as a psychiatric comparison group. Because, among experts, there was considered to be no overlap between the two types of disorders, ADHD was thought to be the perfect control condition.

Much to our surprise we later discovered, while recruiting children for these studies, that a sizable number of kids had to be excluded from participating because they did, in fact, have both an anxiety disorder and ADHD. Around this time other researchers also began to arrive at the same conclusion: ADHD and anxiety disorders can co-occur.

The bottom line for you is that it's possible your child has both of these problems. If you suspect this is the case, you really should get the opinion of a professional who has expertise in diagnosing these disorders in children. Since effective treatments for anxiety disorders and ADHD are not the same, it's important for you to know for sure whether your child has one, the other, or both of these problems.

Depression

Before we get into a discussion of depression in children, I want to mention that true, clinical depression is pretty rare—much rarer than ADHD (which always first makes its appearance in childhood)—in children prior to the onset of puberty. Thus, your elementary-school-age child is unlikely to be experiencing depression, unless, of course, he or she already has entered puberty. (Kids with a preadolescent history of anxiety disorder, though, may be at an increased risk of developing depression during their teenage years, an issue that will be discussed later, in Part II.)

Depression primarily is a disturbance of *mood*. Leslie, a fifth grader who is depressed, feels sad and has frequent crying spells for no apparent reason. Eight-year-old Edward doesn't cry, but he looks "down" most of the time, with his head and shoulders stooped over. He also tells his dad that he feels unhappy a lot of the time.

Depressed kids can have an irritable rather than a sad mood. Sophie, age ten, is described by her mother as being "touchy" and always having "a chip on her shoulder." Gene, a sixth-grade student who is depressed, has angry outbursts many times a day, often yelling at his friends, family, and teachers. He also sometimes has "rage reactions"—punching his fist through his bedroom wall and throwing and breaking objects.

Children with anxiety disorders are not (unless they also are depressed) consistently sad. On the other hand, it's not unusual for an anxious child to be irritable. When irritability occurs in kids with anxiety disorders, it generally is not as pervasive as it is with depressed children. It also doesn't result in the extreme behaviors (such as Gene's destruction of property) sometimes seen in depressed kids.

Although a mood problem is an essential feature of depression, to have this disorder your child must have a cluster of symptoms that includes sadness or irritability along with several others. Symptoms that are characteristic of depression include loss of interest or pleasure in usual activities, changes in appetite and/or weight, changes in sleep, trouble with attention and concentration ("thinking"), feelings of worthlessness or guilt, and, in severe cases, suicidal thoughts or acts or wishes to be dead.

Anxious children do not lose interest in their activities as depressed children do. Your anxious child may be afraid, at times, to participate in certain activities and, as a result, attempt to avoid them, but this is not because he or she lacks interest, energy, or motivation, as is the case with depression. For example, Deidre, a ten-year-old with social phobia, said to her mom, "I don't want to take piano lessons anymore." When her mother questioned her about this, it came out that Deidre had "performance anxiety" about the recitals she knew she would have to participate in.

Depressed children frequently show dramatic and persistent changes in their appetite (and weight) and sleep. Anxious children also sometimes show changes in their eating or sleep patterns, but when these symptoms occur they usually are not consistent. They are linked to specific, anxiety-producing situations.

Yvonne, a nine-year-old with separation anxiety disorder and a fear of going to school, refuses to eat breakfast on school mornings. Her stomach is so upset she's afraid she'll throw up if she eats. On weekends, school holidays, and vacations—when she doesn't have to go to school—Yvonne's appetite for breakfast is just fine.

Anxious children may have difficulty falling asleep on nights before events that make them nervous. Eleven-year-old Alison has trouble going to sleep the evening before a big test at school. Jonathan, who, like Yvonne, has anxiety about leaving home and going to school, has difficulty falling asleep on school nights. He has no trouble with his sleep on evenings of days when school is not in session.

One other difference between the appetite and sleep problems of anxious and depressed children should be mentioned. Depressed children can have problematic *increases*, instead of decreases, in their food intake and sleep time ("hypersomnia"). While anxious children can show an increase in appetite (and weight gain) as a result of their anxiety, this is much less common than a loss of appetite. Excessive sleeping also is rarely seen in anxious children.

If your child becomes depressed, he or she may develop difficulties with attention and concentration, or "trouble thinking," which can result in declining academic performance. While children with anxiety disorders also may, at times, have a problem with the ability to pay attention or concentrate (as I talked about earlier during our discussion of ADHD), it usually is not severe enough to affect their grades.

Depressed children can have extreme feelings of guilt or worthlessness. They blame themselves for things that are not their fault and tend to put themselves down. Because they're feeling so bad, they may have recurring thoughts of death or of hurting themselves or actually try to hurt themselves.

Children with anxiety disorders may "threaten suicide" or proclaim they wish they were dead. This almost always is an attempt to get an adult (a parent, a teacher) to let them out of doing something that causes anxiety—they don't really want to be dead. Kids with anxiety disorders virtually never intentionally try to hurt themselves. Unfortunately, the same cannot be said for depressed children.

If you suspect your child might be depressed, please seek immediate professional assistance. Depression is not something you, as a parent, should handle on your own. It's a serious—sometimes fatal—condition that can require the use of medication and psychological interventions that can be administered only by qualified doctors.

After reading this chapter you should have a pretty good idea of which disorder—or disorders—your child is experiencing. Later, in Part II, when we get into each of the anxiety disorders in much more detail, we'll talk about specific things you can do to help your child with these different problems.

But before we turn to that, let's consider some of the causes of childhood anxiety disorders. If your son or daughter has an anxiety disorder, you're probably wondering how he or she got that way.

3 NATURE OR NURTURE?
The Causes of Childhood Anxiety Disorders

Eight-year-old Connor has just been diagnosed with an anxiety disorder, and his parents feel responsible. "Was it something we did wrong?" they want to know.

Connor's mom is concerned that her overprotective nature may be at fault—she's always telling Connor "Be careful!" and keeps him from doing things that other parents seem to be okay with. She also wonders whether Connor's hospitalization last year (he had complications after a tonsillectomy) could have something to do with his developing an anxiety problem. Connor's dad has his share of guilty feelings too. "Nervous problems" run on his side of the family, and he's worried he may have passed them on to his son.

Why does Connor have an anxiety disorder? Are any—or all—of these things to blame?

Like Connor's parents, you're probably wondering why your child has an anxiety disorder. Like them, you also may blame yourself, asking *"What did I do wrong?"*

But as you'll see in this chapter, many factors can contribute to the development of a childhood anxiety problem, some having to do with a child's relatives and others having nothing at all to do with the family.

Actually, most childhood anxiety disorders occur in the presence of *multiple precipitating factors* or contributory agents—not a single cause. And to complicate things further, the factors that lead to an anxiety disorder in one child often are completely different from

Most childhood anxiety disorders have multiple causes. It's very unusual for a single factor to be at fault.

those that cause an anxiety disorder in another child—even when kids have the *exact same type* of anxiety disorder!

Both Jade and Grace have separation anxiety disorder. Jade's began the fall she started kindergarten and shortly after her nanny—whom she was very attached to—left to take another position. For Grace, though, there didn't seem to be any specific situations linked to the onset of her anxiety disorder. However, her mother recalls having a problem with separation anxiety herself when she was a child. She also admits that the way she is raising Grace tends to be on the overprotective side.

To further complicate matters, even when it seems there is a single circumstance that leads to an anxiety disorder in one child, the same situation can have a different outcome in another child. As neighbors, Darius and Zack were exposed to the same traumatic event. Both of their homes were destroyed by a hurricane last year, but only Zack went on to develop posttraumatic stress disorder. As another example, Ethan and Madison, both eight-year-olds, have parents with obsessive–compulsive disorder. Only Ethan, though, is showing the problem.

In reality, because of the diverse and complex causes of childhood anxiety disorders, and the fact that children have different outcomes with similar histories, you may never know for sure what led to your child's developing an anxiety problem. However, that being said, learning about the different causes of anxiety can help you and your child in another way. It can help you identify things that are contributing to your child's situation *right now*. Then you'll be in a position to make changes that can alter your child's life—now and in the future.

Vince's mom read this chapter and discovered that her son's love of a certain soda pop—one with an extremely high caffeine content—might be playing a role in his anxiety problem. Once she learned about the relationship between caffeine and anxiety, she took immediate action. She put Vince on a caffeine-free diet and was amazed at the rapid improvement in his symptoms.

Trista's father recently has been promoted and is getting a big raise. The family is considering moving to a larger, nicer home across town, but this would mean their daughter, a third grader with an anxiety problem, would have to change schools. After reading this chapter, Trista's parents are concerned that the stress of changing schools might worsen her anxiety. They're now considering postponing the move to when she enters junior high, since she'll have to adjust to a new school then anyway.

Ten-year-old Hillary has always been a skinny child. Thyroid problems—particularly, hyperthyroidism (a "too fast" metabolism that can produce anxiety symptoms)—run in her family, but her mom and dad didn't think someone Hillary's age could have this medical condition. After reading this chapter they suspected their daughter's anxiety symptoms could be due, at least in part, to a thyroid problem. A visit to a pediatric endocrinologist got Hillary properly diagnosed and treated for her metabolic disorder. Her anxiety then improved dramatically.

Heredity versus Environment

When we talk about the multiple potential causes of anxiety disorders in children, it's helpful to make a distinction between *hereditary* causes, present at birth, and *environmental* causes, which influence or affect your child *after* birth.

Hereditary variables are "innate" in your child and are the result of genetic material that has been passed down. (Sometimes conditions children are born with are *congenital*—a result of circumstances that arise during the course of pregnancy, rather than from genes. But for the purpose of this chapter, just to simplify things, we'll include congenital causes together with hereditary factors.)

Environmental factors include events that happen to your child anytime after birth (for example, five days, five months, or five years). Some that can contribute to the development of anxiety disorders include experiencing a trauma, being exposed to certain drugs or substances, or being raised with a particular type of parenting style.

Stressful Life Events

Mental health professionals have long recognized that stressful life events often precede the onset of childhood psychiatric disorders, including anxiety disorders.

Stressful situations your child may have experienced are included in the Children's Life Events checklist on the facing page. By completing it you'll get an understanding of the life situations that may have contributed to your child's problem.

If you take a close look at the events listed, you'll see that most of them fall into one of two general categories. The first category includes events when there is an actual or perceived loss of someone a child is very attached to.

Amelia's mom and dad are getting a divorce. After her dad moved out, Amelia started biting her nails and having nightmares. Eight-year-old Rory became afraid to be away from his mom shortly after his "pap-pap" (grandfather) passed away. When her mom had to stay in the hospital (because her brother was delivered by cesarean), Jena became scared to sleep alone in her room.

A child also can experience a sense of separation and loss in circumstances that are less obvious than the ones I just mentioned. For example, parents can be present in their households but emotionally or physically distant or unavailable to their children. This can happen with moms or dads who have chronic or disabling physical or mental illnesses or substance abuse problems. Parents who have to travel extensively for their jobs also may be perceived of as "removed" by their kids.

The second category of events in the checklist focuses on situations where there has been a major change in a child's immediate, physical environment. A new home, new neighborhood, or new school can create anxiety and contribute to a child's developing an anxiety problem.

Moving even without changing schools can be stressful. When eleven-year-old Rubin's family moved, he became very anxious even though he didn't have to change schools. When I saw Rubin, he was visibly jumpy and upset. With watery eyes he told me he was uncomfortable in the new home and new neighborhood—"I don't like my new room," he said, and "There are no kids in this neighborhood!"

Children's Life Events

1. _____   Death of a parent

2. _____   Death of a brother or sister

3. _____   Death of a grandparent

4. _____   Parents separate or divorce

5. _____   Marriage of parent to stepparent

6. _____   Child hospitalized for serious illness or accident

7. _____   Parent or sibling hospitalized for serious illness or accident

8. _____   Move to a new home

9. _____   Change of schools

10. _____   Brother or sister leaving home

11. _____   Change in parent's job requiring more time away from home

12. _____   Child rejected by peers

13. _____   Failing a grade or being suspended from school

14. _____   Discovery of being adopted

15. _____   Birth of a brother or sister

16. _____   A new adult—stepparent, grandparent—or another child (stepchild, foster child, cousin) moving in

17. _____   Death of child's close friend

18. _____   Separation from family for two weeks or more for any reason

19. _____   Change in family's financial circumstances

20. _____   Any type of highly traumatic event (see Chapter 2, page 41, for specific examples)

When children enter a new school, even if they haven't moved, because their parents decide to change their schools or kids are making the transition from preschool to elementary school or elementary to middle school, they may have difficulty making the adjustment and begin showing signs of anxiety.

When Carly's family decided to take her out of public school and put her in a private elementary school, rather than being pleased, she was panicked. She didn't know anyone at the new school! Who would sit with her at lunch? Who would play with her at recess? What if she didn't like her new teacher?

Because of her discomfort, it was several months before Carly began speaking to the other kids. Even now, a year later, she has great difficulty raising her hand when the teacher asks the class a question. Changing schools—at least in the short run—did not enhance Carly's education. The anxiety it caused her interfered with any potential benefits the new school might offer.

Although things didn't work out well for Carly, I'm not suggesting that a change in schools always has a negative result. To the contrary, the right child–school match can make a world of difference for a child. But when some kids, like Carly, leave what they are accustomed to—their friends, their teacher, even their school building—making the change ends up being too difficult for them.

The last life experience listed in the Children's Life Events checklist includes highly traumatic situations, like the ones described in Chapter 2 when we talked about posttraumatic stress disorder. As you know from that discussion, exposure to an extremely traumatic event (like being the victim of a natural disaster, such as a devastating hurricane or flood, or suffering physical or sexual abuse)—even on a one-time basis—can create extreme anxiety reactions in children.

Sometimes children experience events that are not traumatic enough to produce posttraumatic stress disorder but cause enough of an impact that they create phobias. Even though nobody got hurt, Kirsten developed a fear of riding in cars after she was in an automobile accident with her mom. Richard refused to ride in elevators after he and his father got stuck in one at his dad's office. Sierra thought it would be funny to lock her sister in the hall closet for a few minutes. Not only was it not funny, but her sister then started having panic attacks whenever she was in small or confined places.

Does Anxiety Run in Families?

Research shows that anxiety disorders tend to run in families. Children with anxiety disorders are more likely to have biological relatives with anxiety disorders than kids who don't have anxiety disorders. As you will soon see, however, *more likely to* doesn't mean that all children with anxiety problems have family members with anxiety disorders (or that your child does). It just means that it happens more often than would be expected to occur by chance.

Although a number of studies have focused on this topic, I want to discuss one by our research group because it remains, to my knowledge, the largest and most scientifically rigorous investigation in this area conducted to date.

Almost one hundred children with anxiety disorders, who came from the Child and Adolescent Anxiety Disorder Clinic at the University of Pittsburgh School of Medicine, participated in this study along with their families. Each of the children's immediate family members—their mothers, fathers, and full siblings—were given lengthy, detailed psychiatric interviews. From the children's parents we also obtained information about extended relatives—the children's maternal and paternal aunts, uncles, grandparents, and half-siblings.

The same procedure was used with the families of two other comparison groups of children—a group of kids with other types of psychiatric disorders but no anxiety disorders (from another clinic at the medical center), and a normal group of children from the community, who had no history of any type of psychiatric disorder. In total, 239 children took part in our study and information was obtained on thousands of their biological relatives.

If the premise of our study was correct—that anxiety disorders run in the families of children with these disorders—we would expect higher rates of anxiety disorders in the relatives of the anxious kids than in the relatives in both of the other two groups of children. In fact our results showed that:

- *Over one-third of the close relatives of children with anxiety disorders also had anxiety disorders.* This was significantly higher than the rates for the other two groups of relatives.
- *The same pattern did not hold true for more distant relatives.* While the extended relatives of both the children with anxiety and with other psychiatric disorders had higher rates of anxiety disorders than the normal group, the rates for the two groups with disorders did not differ.

> **Over one-third of the close relatives of kids with anxiety disorders also have anxiety disorders.**

Why did we get the expected results for the children's immediate but not extended relatives? It's possible this was because of the different methods we used to evaluate psychiatric disorders in the two groups. As you'll recall, the children's parents and siblings were interviewed directly about themselves, but information on more distant relatives was obtained secondhand—from the children's parents. Results for extended family members, then, might not be accurate because of the less exacting procedure that was used.

Another way of looking at our findings is to consider that the presence of anxiety disorders is significant in the children's close relatives—the ones they live with—but not their distant or extended family members because the key factor at work here is environmental, not genetic. This would mean that kids develop anxiety disorders because of repeated (environmental) exposure to an immediate family member who has an anxiety problem, not because they inherit genes for an anxiety disorder.

Actually, an additional analysis conducted on our data could be interpreted as giving some support for this idea. When we looked at anxiety disorders *within* individual families, in the parents of children with anxiety-disorders rather than *across* families (that is, for the group of kids as a whole), we found that two-thirds of the children had at least one parent who had an anxiety disorder.

Before you become alarmed, let me emphasize that many parents with anxiety disorders have children who *do not* also develop anxiety disorders. The study we just discussed (and others like it) used what is referred to as the "bottom up" method—that's where children with anxiety disorders are identified and then their relatives are looked at to see if they also have anxiety problems. When you use this approach, you get *much higher* figures than if you use the approach—the "top down" method—where parents with anxiety disorders are identified and then *their children* are examined to see if they too have anxiety problems.

Again, please be assured, if you or your spouse has an anxiety disorder, this does not mean that all—or any—of your children will have anxiety problems! However, with that being said, what should you do if you (or your spouse) happen to fall into this group?

If you know, or suspect, that you have an anxiety disorder, it probably would be a good idea to get some help with this. This may mean availing yourself of some of the many wonderful self-help books for anxiety that are on the market or even getting professional help. Although no one wants to have an anxiety problem, the good news is that anxiety disorders are probably the most readily, successfully treated of all psychiatric problems, given, of course, that the appropriate intervention techniques are used (many of which you will find in Part II of this book).

The Specificity of Anxiety Disorders within Families

Anxiety disorders tend to run in families, but do they run true to form? Do relatives in the same family have the same specific type of anxiety disorder?

Nine-year-old Spence has obsessive–compulsive disorder. His father, his father's sister (Spence's paternal aunt), and his dad's own father (Spence's paternal grandfather) also have obsessive–compulsive disorder. Is this just a coincidence, or does this anxiety disorder affect families in this way?

On the other hand, Meagan, a fifth grader with generalized anxiety disorder, shows a different family picture. Although a number of her relatives have anxiety disorders, none of them have the same one she has.

Spence's case suggests that the same specific type of anxiety disorder occurs within families, while Meagan's family situation leads us to believe otherwise. Actually, the results from the study I just discussed addressed this issue and showed that both scenarios—that seen in Spence's and in Meagan's families—take place. Which way things turn out depends on which anxiety disorder you are talking about.

Our study showed that kids with obsessive–compulsive disorder are more likely to have relatives with obsessive–compulsive disorder than kids with other types of anxiety disorders. Children with other anxiety disorders may have family members with anxiety disorders, but not necessarily the same ones they have.

> **With the exception of obsessive–compulsive disorder, the <u>same exact</u> anxiety disorders don't usually appear in children and their family members.**

As you'll see in the next section, genetic research has shown the same specificity for obsessive–compulsive disorder that we found, suggesting it may have the strongest hereditary component of all of the individual anxiety disorders.

The Genetic Contribution

Family studies like the one I just talked about can tell you that anxiety disorders run in families, but they do not tell you whether this happens because of genes, the family environment (for example, the way parents interact with their children), or some combination of the two. Moreover, it's possible that the cause—genetic or environmental—is not the same for different anxiety disorders.

Genetic research strategies that separate hereditary from environmental influences are used to assess the extent to which genes contribute to anxiety disorders. In "twin research," rates of anxiety disorders are compared for identical twins (who share 100 percent of their genes) and fraternal twins (who share only 50 percent of their genes—the same as for two nontwin siblings). "Adoption studies," another research strategy used among geneticists, tease out environmental factors from purely hereditary ones in a different way. They compare rates of anxiety disorders in individuals "at risk" for developing an anxiety disorder (because many of their biological relatives already have anxiety disorders) who are raised either with or apart from their biological parents. More recent methodological advancements also now allow researchers to take blood samples and look directly at genetic material.

The genetic research conducted thus far overall shows there is an inherited component to anxiety disorders but that it's limited. By *limited* I mean that the strength of the genetic contribution, at least based on the present evidence, is considerably less than for other types of psychiatric disorders (for example, bipolar disorder or schizophrenia). In addition, the strength of the genetic contribution varies for the different, specific anxiety disorders.

When considering the anxiety disorders preadolescent children experience, obsessive–compulsive disorder and, to a lesser extent, social anxiety disorder are most influenced by genetic factors. Post-traumatic stress disorder and generalized anxiety disorder seem to be the least affected by genes.

> **Obsessive–compulsive disorder and, to a lesser extent, social anxiety disorder are most influenced by genes.**

Do you remember from our study the overall rate of anxiety disorders—the group percentage—for the close relatives of children with anxiety disorders? It was slightly over one-third. Although this was a significant finding, it's important to keep in mind that this percentage wasn't as high as what would have been expected *if* the development of anxiety disorders truly were determined primarily or solely by genes.

The Anxious Temperament

Is it possible that genetic studies haven't come up with very impressive results because in looking for anxiety *disorders* something else that is being passed on is being overlooked? This is the argument put forth by researchers who specialize in the area of infant temperament.

Given this book is about anxiety disorders, it's appropriate to talk about one particular type of temperament—"the anxious temperament." The anxious temperament, as is true for other temperament styles, is first observed right after birth but persists, too, as children get older.

Newborns and infants who are considered "colicky"—who seem to be constantly crying and are hard, if not impossible, to soothe—often have anxious temperaments. Toddlers and preschoolers who have strong startle responses (really jump when they hear or see something unexpected), are very hesitant to enter new situations, and have a hard time getting used to or "adjusted" to these new situations may have anxious temperaments.

> **Newborns and infants who are considered "colicky" often have anxious temperaments.**

The anxious temperament is characterized by three things: (1) a high arousal level when "at rest" (not stressed); (2) extreme physiological reactivity to novel stimuli—new objects, people, and situations; and (3) failure to show decreased reactivity to the unfamiliar with repeated exposure over time.

Three-year-old Hailey has an anxious temperament. When her mom took her for her first haircut, her reaction was like someone having surgery without an anesthetic. She was hysterical—screamed and cried nonstop, turned red in the face, and kept trying to get out of the chair. She had the same reaction when her mother took her to be fitted for her first real pair of shoes. Not only does Hailey get frightened and upset in new situations; once she gets that way, it's impossible to get her to calm down. Despite giving her the verbal reassurance and physical closeness that she demands (Hailey has a tendency to cling to her mother), her mom says, "Nothing I do ever seems to work."

Luke's parents want to put him in preschool next fall, but they're concerned he might not be able to handle it. Luke still has trouble separating from his mom when she goes to her part-time job, even though she's been doing this since he was born. Luke also is very uncomfortable with kids his age, even those he's seen every week for the past year at mommy-and-me classes. Luke's mom and dad don't understand why Luke doesn't "get used to" things. "It's like each time is the first time," they say.

Children with anxious temperaments are more prone to acquire fears than children with other types of temperaments. Preliminary research also suggests that having an anxious temperament as a child may increase the likelihood of developing an anxiety disorder later on. As more studies are done on this subject, the relationship between this style of temperament and anxiety disorders will, hopefully, become clearer.

The Powerful Effects of Caffeine

While it's well known that caffeine is widely used by adults, many people don't realize how much is consumed by children. Although children don't typically drink coffee (which is extremely high in caffeine unless it's "decaf"), they eat certain foods and drink other beverages that contain large amounts of caffeine.

Make no mistake about it: caffeine is most certainly a drug and a very potent one at that. It is a central nervous system stimulant, which means that in sufficient quantities it has the potential to produce anxiety symptoms, like jitteriness, nervousness, an elevated heart rate, and sweating. Anxiety-prone children (like kids with anxious temperaments or those who have anxiety disorders that run in their families) and children with anxiety disorders are particularly sensitive to caffeine and can have extreme anxiety reactions—even panic attacks—from relatively low amounts.

An additional problem with caffeine is that it triggers the release of insulin in the body, which ultimately leads to a decreased level of sugar in the blood (a spike and then a plummet). When blood sugar levels drop, children may have hypoglycemic (low blood sugar) reactions that can include anxiety symptoms.

The sidebar on the following page lists the caffeine content of many high-caffeine foods and beverages consumed by children every day. As you can see, certain sodas (including all of the colas, with the exception of those that are "caffeine-free" or have "reduced caffeine"), iced-tea drinks (except those that are herbal or decaffeinated), and chocolate are especially high in caffeine content. Caffeine-free alternatives are available for many of these products, particularly the beverages (for example, decaf or naturally caffeine-free sodas, herbal or decaffeinated teas).

While I know it can be hard to get your child to give up a favorite beverage (and even harder to let go of chocolate), keeping these things out of your home and replacing them with no- or low-caffeine products will certainly help. Enlisting the assistance of other adults

Caffeine Content of Foods and Beverages

Product	Caffeine (milligrams)
Soda	
Mountain Dew (12 ounces)	55
Coca-Cola (12 ounces)	45
Dr. Pepper (12 ounces)	41
Sunkist Orange Soda (12 ounces)	40
Pepsi (12 ounces)	37
Tea	
Snapple iced tea (16 ounces)	48
Lipton tea (8 ounces)	38
Chocolate	
Hershey's Special Dark chocolate bar (1.5 ounces)	31
Hershey's Milk Chocolate bar (1.5 ounces)	10
Hot chocolate (8 ounces)	5

who will be supervising your child when you're not around—your child's teacher, parents of kids your child has play dates with—is also a good idea. If you explain to them the importance of your child's avoiding caffeine, most people will be happy to help you with this. Parents also may be able to motivate their children to steer away from "the bad stuff" when they're not there to police them if they explain— in a way that the child will understand—that certain foods and drinks bring on the anxiety symptoms they want to get rid of.

When Elise's parents brought her to see me, they were at the end of their rope. Elise had become "impossible" lately—nervous, irritable, moody, anxious about going places. Even though Elise had always had an anxious tendency, in the last few months she'd gotten much worse. When I questioned her folks about her diet, I discovered that Elise, although only eleven, recently had begun going with Dad to Starbucks and drinking coffee almost every day when her father picked her up from school. To make matters even worse, Elise's favorite soda was cola, which is loaded with caffeine. Elise also confided that she was a chocoholic—she regularly ate chocolate candy, chocolate chip cookies, and chocolate ice cream.

During my discussions with Elise and her parents I explained to them that caffeine might be to blame for Elise's worsening anxiety. I gave them a copy of the chart on the facing page, and we came up with caffeine-free alternatives that Elise said she would be okay with. When the family returned in two weeks, they were happy to report that Elise was back to her old self. A simple change in diet had produced a marked change in Elise's emotional state. (As with Elise, in my practice I've found that kids, even fairly young ones, are surprisingly cooperative with dietary restrictions and changes once they're convinced that they will be of help.)

Medical Problems

A number of medical conditions can cause, contribute to, or mimic anxiety disorders in children. They are listed in the sidebar on the following page.

The medical problem that probably is most commonly singled out as causing anxiety problems is hyperthyroidism, which basically is a "too fast" metabolism. Interestingly, however, physicians who specialize in thyroid dysfunction recently have acknowledged that low thyroid—*hypo*thyroidism—also can be associated with anxiety. To compound matters, the drugs used to treat hypothyroidism frequently produce anxiety symptoms as side effects.

Earlier we talked about how caffeine can trigger hypoglycemic reactions, which often have anxiety as a component. But even children who are on caffeine-restricted diets can become hypoglycemic. Skipping meals, going a long period of time between meals (without snacks), or having sugary snacks in place of meals all can produce low blood sugar.

Medical Conditions
That Can Produce Anxiety Symptoms

Endocrine and metabolic disorders
  Hypo- and hyperthyroidism
  Adrenal dysfunction (Addison's disease and Cushing's syndrome)
  Hypoglycemia
  Diabetes

Neurological disorders
  Epilepsy
  Head injury
  Postconcussive syndrome

Inner ear disturbances (that result in a disturbance of balance)

Respiratory conditions
  Allergies
  Asthma
  Hyperventilation syndrome

Heart problems
  Cardiac arrhythmias
  Mitral valve prolapse

Certain vitamin and mineral deficiencies

Food allergies and intolerances

Chemical sensitivities and exposure to environmental toxins

Often overlooked is the contribution of allergic reactions and chemical sensitivities to anxiety problems. Common environmental (inhalant) allergies, including reactions to, for instance, pet dander, mold, dust, or pollen, as well as food allergies—for example, to wheat, corn, soy, milk, citrus, or beef—can produce anxiety symptoms. If your child appears to suffer from seasonal or chronic respiratory (stuffy nose, sneezing) or skin problems (hives, eczema, unexplained rashes), you should consider taking him or her to a pediatric allergist to check things out.

There are several forms of allergy testing (through the blood or the skin) that can help identify what specific things your child is allergic to. However, if you don't want to go this route (it can be expensive), you can try keeping a log. Note when your child is exposed to things you suspect may be causing a problem and then record his or her reactions. Although this can be time-consuming, it's a good way to identify allergy problems that are not clearly obvious (obvious being, for example, watery eyes and sneezing whenever your child is around cats).

Exposures to chemicals—whether ingested (for instance, medications, preservatives, dyes, artificial flavorings), inhaled (like pesticides, car exhaust, cigarette smoke, fragrances), or topical (in certain soaps, creams, and detergents)—have the potential, in susceptible children, to trigger anxietylike reactions. Problems with chemicals don't always show up on testing because they frequently aren't true allergic reactions but rather are "sensitivities." Probably the best way to approach these is to use the log approach. In this way you can identify chemicals you suspect are causing your child's problem, then eliminate or reduce exposure to them.

Are You Teaching Your Child to Be Anxious?

Earlier I briefly mentioned that parents' own anxiety problems may play a role in their children's developing anxiety disorders. In fact children can learn to be anxious through behaviors—both verbal and nonverbal—that their parents display. This can happen even with moms or dads who do not have diagnosable anxiety disorders (but it's probably more likely to happen with parents who do).

There are several possible ways that you could, unknowingly and unintentionally, foster anxiety in your child. A major route is through observational learning.

Learning through Observation

Research has shown that children learn from observing and then imitating others. Parents of young children will hardly be surprised by this finding. You watched your child speak his or her first words

("Say *mama!*") and develop simple skills (like clapping hands) in this way.

Children also can learn emotional responses—like fear and anxiety—through observation and imitation. And the closer and more important the person is to the child—as with a parent, for example—the more likely it is that this learning will take place.

Chloe's mom has been afraid of cats as long as she can remember. Although she doesn't want her daughter to have this fear, she can't help how she reacts when she sees a cat. She becomes visibly shaky, grabs Chloe's hand, and gets them away as fast as possible.

By the time she's four, Chloe is reacting to cats like her mom. But Chloe's fear isn't limited to actual encounters with cats. She also gets upset when she sees one in her picture books or on the cartoons on TV. Unfortunately Chloe probably has developed a phobia from observing her mom's fear.

Some parents find they're able to control their reactions and successfully hide their fears from their children. But if, like Chloe's mom, you find you can't, I encourage you to take steps to get rid of your fear. As I mentioned earlier, you can do this with self-help books written for adults with anxiety problems or by seeking professional help or even by using some of the strategies for reducing anxiety contained in Part II of this book.

Reinforcing Fear and Avoidance

The attention of a parent (verbal and physical) is one of the most powerful forms of reinforcement there is for a child. Without realizing it, some parents, in comforting and consoling their children when they exhibit fears, actually strengthen their children's fears rather than helping to reduce them, as is their intention.

Mia has always been somewhat shy. Her mom thought it would be a good idea for her to start taking ballet classes when she turned five so she'd have an opportunity to meet new kids her age. Although Mia initially was excited and looking forward to her first class, when it came time to enter the dance studio she stopped dead in her tracks.

After a lot of encouragement from her mom she did go in, but she felt awkward and uncomfortable with the other little girls, none of whom she knew. After about five minutes, with tears running down her face, she darted out of the classroom and down the hall to the reception area where her mom was waiting. Her mom put her arms around her, hugged her tight, and told her, "It's okay, honey. You don't have to come back here again."

To her credit, Mia's mom was successful in getting her daughter to enter the dance studio. But seeing her daughter reduced to tears, she consoled and comforted her and promised not to push again. Although her mother's response was very sympathetic, it may make it harder for Mia to enter other new social situations in the future.

What could Mia's mother have done that might have turned things around? She could have arranged for Mia to meet some of the other kids who were going to be in her dance class beforehand, so they would be familiar to her by the first class. It also might have helped for Mia to have visited the dance studio ahead of time—to get used to the building, meet her teacher, watch another class in progress to see how things are run—so that the situation as a whole would have been less new to her. Finally, it probably would have been better for Mia's mom to drop her off at the studio and come back for her at the end of class. Most teachers have a lot of experience dealing with children's anxieties. It's a good bet that Mia's ballet instructor might have handled her situation successfully given the chance.

Sometimes parents—particularly those who have a strong fear or anxiety about something themselves—encourage and then reinforce fearful behavior in their children. As an example, look at what this dog-phobic mother says to her daughter as the child approaches the neighbor's dog:

Mother: Honey, don't go near the dog.

(Child responds by retreating from the animal.)

Mother: Good girl.

Although the process at work here is somewhat different from observational learning (the child in this situation isn't watching her mom or dad behave fearfully), this child also is learning to be fearful. Her mother is transferring her own fear on to her daughter by prompting and then rewarding (verbally) avoidance behavior.

The Anxious World View

Some people (frequently those with anxiety disorders) have a way of looking at life and the world at large that emphasizes danger and uncertainty and promotes anxiety. The "anxious world view" is a belief system that can be summarized something like this: "The world is a frightening, scary, and unpredictable place, where bad things often happen."

Parents with this attitude, without meaning to, can teach it to their kids. This is something like observational learning, but in this case the child learns a set of emotional responses and behaviors that are linked together by a common theme—potential danger— rather than developing a problem with a specific situation.

Terrell's dad has an anxious view of the world. He always assumes the worst is going to happen. When the family travels by plane, he insists they split up and go on separate flights. Terrell's mom goes with his sister while Terrell travels with his dad on a different flight that's going to the same place. This way, his father figures, they won't all die if something goes wrong.

Terrell's father also worries about being robbed. He tells his son that he always carries his money in several different places—in his right pants pocket, in a money belt hidden under his clothes, and in the inside pocket of his jacket—so he won't lose it all if he's mugged.

In reading about Terrell's father you may have found yourself understanding his point of view. Especially now, in light of recent world events (like the terrorist attacks on the United States), people's attitudes about potential danger have changed. Parents also are more frightened about the safety of their children. It seems like crimes against children are happening more frequently each day (although it's hard to know whether there really has been an increase in these types of crimes or it just appears so because of the tremendous media attention they receive). Today having an anxious view of the world seems less unreasonable than it did a decade or two ago.

Despite some very real potential dangers in the world we live in today, I think we can agree that it's not healthy or helpful to regard our future and the future of our children as likely filled with catastrophic events. Not only is it not helpful, it probably isn't accurate. Taking a wider historical view of things, catastrophic events really do not happen frequently, certainly not frequently enough to support adopting an overly anxious outlook.

If you think that you (or your spouse) have an overly anxious view of the world, I encourage you to take steps to change this. People can alter their perceptions with certain therapeutic techniques—namely, *cognitive therapy* techniques—many of which, in fact, are described in Part II of this book. There also are other cognitive therapy methods available that aren't used with children. Go to the psychology self-help section of your bookstore or look for a cognitive therapist near you. You'll be doing something positive for yourself and for your child as well.

An Overprotective Parenting Style

Some parents (often ones with an anxious world view) consistently overprotect their children. Although they have the best of intentions, this approach to child rearing can increase a kid's chance of developing an anxiety problem.

Isabelle's mom is overprotective. After watching so many stories on TV about children being kidnapped, she's not comfortable with Isabelle doing things away from home without her. She didn't allow Isabelle to go on the overnight trip with her sixth-grade class even though there were four adult chaperones for the twenty kids who went. She also won't let Isabelle go to the mall or to the movies with her friends.

Clay, a third grader, is upset with how his mom "babies" him. She won't let him participate in sports because she's scared he might get hurt. She also insists on doing things for him—like cutting his meat into little pieces—that he's old enough to do for himself.

Seven-year-old Bethany also has a mother who is overprotective. Bethany's mom has never taken a vacation alone with Bethany's dad because she's not comfortable being away from her kids. She also won't leave them with a real babysitter—it has to be a relative—because she doesn't trust anyone else with her children.

Children who are overprotected—like the children I just described—don't have the opportunities they need to learn how to face and handle life's challenges. As a result they may not mature at the same rate as other kids. Adolescence can be a particularly tough time for them—generating a lot of anxiety because of the new expectations and changes that arise (social, academic, biological). Rather than becoming more independent and autonomous (as is the norm during the teenage years), they may remain close to home and to their families. Unfortunately these kids then keep missing out on experiences that are important for their growth and confidence building.

The questionnaire on the facing page will tell you if—like Isabelle's, Clay's, and Bethany's parents—you have a parenting style that tends to be somewhat overprotective. Try to be objective and also avoid being overly critical of yourself when you fill out this questionnaire. The goal is not to point any fingers of blame but to identify factors contributing to your child's anxiety that you have the power to change. If you respond with a "yes" to three or more of the questions, this probably is a problem area for you.

If you are too overprotective of your child, and you want to change this, there are a number of things you can do. Talking to other parents of children the same age as your child is one way of getting a sense of the age-appropriateness of the rules and limits you set for your child. Observing how other moms and dads behave toward their kids—what they do and don't do for them, how they respond to minor injuries and childhood illnesses, how much they worry about them and how they tolerate separations—gives you additional information about what the norm is. Taking parenting classes or consulting with a professional who is knowledgeable and sensitive to these issues (your child's pediatrician, teacher, or someone in the mental health field) also can be very helpful.

An Overcritical Parenting Style

Parents who are excessively critical of their children—constantly pointing out their flaws and mistakes and rarely praising or rewarding them—may be contributing to their kids' developing anxiety problems.

Cooper's dad is very tough on him. If Cooper comes home with a report card with all A's and one B, his dad ignores the A's and de-

Could You Be an Overprotective Parent?

	Yes	No
Do you worry about your child's safety more than you should or more than makes sense?	☐	☐
Do you keep your child from doing things that other parents of kids your child's age are okay with?	☐	☐
Do you "baby" your child? Do you do things for your child that he or she should be able to do for him- or herself?	☐	☐
Do you have a lot of trouble being separated from your child?	☐	☐
When you are not with your child, do you often worry that something bad might happen?	☐	☐
When your child wants to avoid a situation (one that isn't dangerous or problematic) because he or she feels frightened or uncomfortable, do you readily "give in"?	☐	☐
Do you overreact when your child has minor aches, pains, or injuries or common childhood illnesses?	☐	☐

FROM *HELP FOR WORRIED KIDS* BY CYNTHIA G. LAST. COPYRIGHT 2006 BY CYNTHIA G. LAST.

mands to know "Why'd you get the B?" When they play touch football together and Cooper misses a catch, his dad gets angry and shouts, "You play like a girl!" After Cooper tried out a new way of doing his hair (spiked with gel, like his friends do), his father told him he looked ridiculous.

Rosemary's mom is not quite as obvious as Cooper's dad, but she also is overly critical of her child. When Rosemary picked out a dress for her elementary school graduation that wasn't her mom's choice, her mother frowned and asked, "Do you *really* like that?" At her graduation party Rosemary enthusiastically pointed out the boy she has a crush on. To her disappointment her mother responded by saying, "Don't you think he's kind of funny looking?"

Children who have an overly critical mom or dad often become hypervigilant ("on alert"), preparing themselves for the hurtful comments they expect to receive. They may worry excessively about making mistakes (and be very hard on themselves when they think they've made one) in one particular or several areas, such as in social situations, with their schoolwork, or in how they perform in their hobbies and recreational activities. To avoid making mistakes and the criticism this brings, they may become perfectionists or even develop compulsive checking rituals (anxiety symptoms, as you'll see in Part II, that are common in certain anxiety disorders).

Some parents are overly critical of their children because that's how they were raised. They are repeating behaviors that are familiar to them, usually not realizing how damaging it is to their kids. For other parents their excessive negativity stems from emotional problems (often depression) they're experiencing.

If Cooper's dad had gotten help for his depression, he might have been more positive toward his son. And if Rosemary's mom had been aware that she was behaving toward her daughter just like her mom had toward her, she might have done something about it. Unfortunately for both of these children, neither of these things happened.

Your situation can be different. Having read this you can take a look at yourself and determine whether you have a problem like this. Again, the point in determining whether your parenting style is overcritical is not to make you feel guilty but to help you recognize behavior that you may not be fully aware of. Many parents whose style is somewhat overcritical have the best of intentions for their kids; all they want is to help them learn to work hard and do their best. If you think there's a chance that you tend to go overboard in this endeavor, please consider the different avenues for change that I've talked about throughout this chapter. Both you and your child will reap the rewards.

Over-the-Counter and Prescription Medications

Certain over-the-counter medications can cause anxiety symptoms as side effects. For example, you should be aware that pseudoephedrine, a common ingredient (used as a decongestant) in many cold and allergy products manufactured for children, has the ability to cause anxiety reactions, particularly in kids who are anxiety-prone. Also, some kids have anxious or agitated reactions, rather than the more typical sedation effect, to over-the-counter antihistamines (if you read the small print on the back of the box, you'll see this mentioned as a possible reaction in children).

Prescription medications, as mentioned before about thyroid replacement drugs, sometimes produce anxiety symptoms. In fact psychiatric drugs, including ones used for the treatment of anxiety disorders in children, can, paradoxically, increase rather than decrease anxiety. Sometimes this is only temporary, until the child has gotten used to the medication. Other times it means that the child's psychiatrist (or other treating physician) needs to consider using a different drug.

Just as the use of certain drugs can elicit anxiety symptoms, the discontinuation of certain medications, especially after they've been used for some time, can produce an anxiety reaction, particularly if the substance is withdrawn abruptly. Certain psychiatric drugs are well known for this. As an example, benzodiazepines (a class of antianxiety medications) must be tapered slowly (if the child has been on a substantial dose for a prolonged period of time) to avoid "withdrawal symptoms" that often include anxiety. Some of the selective serotonin reuptake inhibitors, or SSRIs, which also are frequently used by psychiatrists to treat childhood anxiety disorders, can have a "discontinuation syndrome" associated with their withdrawal. The syndrome produces anxiety symptoms that can be even worse than the child's original condition.

Please do not take my cautionary remarks about prescription medications, including psychiatric drugs, to mean that I don't support their use. While an in-depth discussion of the psychopharmacological treatment of anxiety disorders is beyond the scope of this book, suffice it to say that many children, including those with anxiety disorders, have been helped enormously through the advances made in this area. As an informed parent, though, I think you should be aware that for certain kids some of these drugs can induce—through their administration or termination—the very problem you are trying to get rid of.

Parents often spend a great deal of time trying to figure out why their sons and daughters have anxiety disorders. As I said at the beginning of this chapter, because there are so many possible contributors, it's hard to know for sure what led to the development of an anxiety disorder in a particular child.

If you aren't able to identify the factors that led to your child's developing a problem with anxiety, you shouldn't be overly concerned. As you'll see in Part II, successfully dealing with childhood anxiety disorders generally does not rely on understanding causes. Once you know what the problem is—a phobia, separation anxiety, or obsessive–compulsive disorder, for example—what you need to do to help your child is pretty straightforward.

Let's get to this now.

PART II

The Anxiety Disorders of Childhood

4 "WILL YOU STILL BE THERE TOMORROW?"
Separation Anxiety Disorder

The night before he's supposed to leave for camp Hunter tells his dad, "I can't go." Hunter has never been away from his parents for more than a couple of nights. To tell the truth, he really doesn't like—isn't comfortable—being away from home even when he's with his mom and dad, like when they went on vacation last summer. Now he's expected to be away from home and his parents for four whole weeks and he's overwhelmed with fear.

At ten Hunter's folks think he should be able to handle going to camp, but he's pleading to stay home. Should they make him go? Or would it be better to wait till he's older?

In Chapter 1 we talked about the fact that almost all kids go through a period between six months and two and a half years when they're scared of being apart from their moms. Even after two and a half it still can be normal for kids to have trouble separating at times, like when they begin day care or preschool. The anxiety usually continues for a few days or, at most, a week or two and doesn't have a major or long-lasting effect on kids or their families.

It's a different story, though, when children are past the usual age for separation anxiety and continue to have severe distress during separations. When anxiety like this goes on for weeks or even months and interferes with your child's ability to do things expected of kids his or her age, it's a sign that your child may have separation anxiety disorder.

While normal separation anxiety goes away on its own as your child matures, separation anxiety *disorder* usually does not. This particular anxiety disorder tends to be episodic: it has distinct periods when it's present and those when it's absent, so when you think your child has bypassed the problem you may be unpleasantly surprised to find it recur, especially during times of stress or transition. Also, many children who suffer from separation anxiety disorder are at increased risk of developing other anxiety disorders during adolescence and early adulthood. So by addressing your child's problem now you'll not only be helping your son or daughter feel better (and function better) at this time; you'll be giving him or her a chance for a better future.

Of all the childhood anxiety disorders, separation anxiety disorder is the most common. Fortunately, though, when handled correctly it usually is relatively easy to get rid of. Later on we'll discuss practical things you can do to help your child overcome the fear of separation. But first let's talk more about separation anxiety disorder and how to know for sure if your child has this problem.

Diagnosing Separation Anxiety Disorder

Although separation anxiety disorder has been described in the psychiatric and psychological literature since the 1950s, it was not until 1980, with the American Psychiatric Association's publication of the third edition of the *Diagnostic and Statistic Manual of Mental Disorders* (the classification system used to diagnose psychiatric disorders in the United States), that it was given diagnostic status and officially recognized as a childhood anxiety disorder.

How separation anxiety disorder has been defined in the DSM has changed somewhat since that time, but the essential features remain pretty much the same. I've listed the symptoms of the disorder in the sidebar on the facing page. All of the symptoms are indications of developmentally inappropriate, persistent, and excessive anxiety about separating from a major attachment figure (usually a parent) or from home.

As you can see, eight symptoms are described, but only three are needed for your child to be diagnosed with this anxiety disorder. Also, for a diagnosis of separation anxiety disorder, the three (or more) symptoms your child has must have gone on for at least four weeks.

The "cardinal" feature of separation anxiety disorder is the distress children have when anticipating or experiencing a separation. Some kids become distressed about separations that involve being away from home (even if they're with their parents), while others have problems when they have to be apart from a major attachment figure (either being at home or leaving home without the person) or in both types of situations. (As you'll remember from Chapter 2, a major attachment figure can be *anyone* a child is extremely attached to. But because in most instances this person is a child's mother, and to simplify things, I'll assume this is the case in much of what I say in this chapter.)

Separation-related distress is shown in different ways. When six-

Symptoms of Separation Anxiety Disorder

To be diagnosed with this disorder, the child must have at least three of these symptoms:

- Becomes extremely distressed when separated from someone the child is extremely attached to (usually a parent) or from the home or when anticipating separation.

- Worries excessively about losing a person (usually a parent) the child is extremely attached to or about that person being harmed.

- Worries excessively that some terrible event will happen to the child that will separate him or her from someone the child is extremely attached to (usually a parent) or from home.

- Doesn't want to or won't go to school or other places (without a parent) because of separation fears.

- Doesn't want to or won't be at home without someone the child is extremely attached to (usually a parent) because of separation fears.

- Doesn't want to or won't go to sleep without being near someone the child is extremely attached to (usually a parent) *or* sleep away from home.

- Has recurring nightmares about being separated (like about being kidnapped or killed).

- Complains of feeling sick when faced with separation.

year-old Claudia's mom tries to leave her at home with a babysitter, her daughter clings to her leg and won't let go. Heidi, age ten, also gets upset at being left at home, but since she's older she uses her verbal abilities to try to persuade her mom to take her along. Adrienne, a fourth grader who is afraid to leave home to go to school, has stomachaches on school mornings. Eleven-year-old Parker, who also has anxiety about going to school, has panic attacks in the classroom and wants to come home.

Children with separation anxiety disorder frequently have worries about something bad happening to them or their parents. Almost every day Anthony, a third grader with separation anxiety, worries that his mom will get into a car accident. Six-year-old Bianca keeps thinking that "something bad" is going to happen to her mom and that she'll never see her again. Cameron, age eight, is scared he's going to get lost and be separated from his mom when he's out with her in large, crowded places, like at the mall or in the supermarket.

Please keep in mind that the worries I just talked about must be *persistent and excessive* to be signs of separation anxiety disorder. As I discussed in Chapter 1, kids who don't have anxiety disorders also sometimes worry about bad things happening to them (particularly about being kidnapped or getting lost) or to their parents. The significance of these worries (that is, whether *you* need to worry about them) depends on how often they occur and how long they've gone on, and, to a lesser degree, their context. For example, if your child starts worrying about being kidnapped while a child abduction case is being highlighted on the news, and it passes in a few days, this isn't indicative of separation anxiety disorder.

A child's reluctance or refusal to go to school or to go other places because of fear of being away from a parent or home is another common symptom of separation anxiety disorder. Casey, a third grader, will go to school only if her mom goes with her and stays in the school building. Eight-year-old Caitlin's parents want to send her to day camp this summer, but she doesn't want to go. She's nervous about being away from home for so many hours, so many days a week. Six-year-old Amelia won't play at the little girl's house next door because she doesn't want to be away from her mom.

Kids also often have fears of being at home without a major attachment figure, or of being home alone if they're old enough to do this. (Parents vary quite a bit on the age at which they consider it appropriate to leave a child alone at home. Besides age they also take into consideration other factors, like whether it's light or dark outside, the length of time the child will be alone, and how far they—the parents—will be from home.) Anxiety being at home without a major attachment figure but with another adult (a babysitter; other adult family members) or older siblings is common for many kids with separation anxiety disorder.

Young children with separation anxiety disorder sometimes have trouble being on a different floor of their house, or even in a different room on the same floor, than their mothers. If your child is like this, he or she may follow you from room to room. Eight-year-old Tova repeatedly calls out to her mom when the two of them are in different rooms, just to make sure she's still there and is "all right."

Sleeping alone in their own rooms or sleeping away from home can be major problems for children with this anxiety disorder. Shannon, who's in the third grade, is scared of sleeping in her room. Night after night she slips down the hall and into her parents' bed, asking if she can sleep with them. Demi, a sixth grader who is much like Hunter (the boy I described at the very beginning of this chapter), is terrified of the idea of going to sleep-away camp. Olivia, age eleven, isn't able to go to sleepovers at her friends' homes. She's too nervous about being away from home overnight.

Younger kids with separation anxiety disorder, particularly between the ages of five and eight, are likely to have recurring nightmares about events involving separation. The bad dreams usually are about being kidnapped or getting lost or about parents being in an accident, getting sick, or dying.

Kids frequently have physical complaints when anticipating or confronting separation. Your child may have stomachaches (or even vomit), or have headaches or pain in other parts of the body before or during separations. Sometimes the complaints are less specific and children just say "I don't feel well" or "I think I'm getting sick." It's important to keep in mind that physical symptoms that have a medical cause (this has to be determined by a physician) are not considered to be part, or an indication of, separation anxiety disorder.

As you will recall, *distress* and *impairment* are topics that were discussed at length in Chapter 1. For your child to be diagnosed with separation anxiety disorder the symptoms he or she has (from the list on page 83) have to be severe enough to cause extreme distress or interfere with the ability to perform age-expected activities, like going to school, participating in other activities away from home, and forming and maintaining friendships. (If your child has separation anxiety symptoms but doesn't meet this criterion, it's probably a subclinical level of separation anxiety, another subject we talked about in the first chapter.)

Do children's ages or gender influence how separation anxiety is expressed? A study our research group conducted in the late 1980s at our Pittsburgh child anxiety clinic, described in *Child Psychiatry and Human Development*, addressed this issue. The results of our study showed that younger kids (ages five through eight) with separation anxiety disorder had more symptoms of the disorder than older kids (ages nine through twelve) diagnosed with the disorder. In fact although the presence of only three symptoms from the list on page 83 is required for the diagnosis, all of the younger children had four or more symptoms. For gender our findings showed no differences between boys and girls—both groups of kids had the same types and number of separation anxiety symptoms.

Younger children with separation anxiety disorder tend to have more symptoms of the disorder than older children.

The Many Faces of Separation Anxiety Disorder

Although the "hallmark" of separation anxiety disorder—fear of being separated from someone the child is extremely attached to or from home—is the same for all children with this problem, the specific way the disorder appears (as we just saw for younger versus older kids) is different for different kids. Since only three of eight symptoms are required for the diagnosis, numerous symptom combinations are possible, all of which would meet the criteria for having this disorder.

Let's now take an in-depth look at four children, all of whom have separation anxiety disorder but are experiencing it in somewhat different ways.

Ashley

At nine Ashley is having difficulty sleeping alone. For months she's been trying to convince her parents to let her sleep in their bed. When her mom makes her go back to her room, she gets very upset and begs to stay, but her mom won't give in. Ashley ends up sleeping on the floor in the hallway right outside her parent's door.

Ashley also is giving her folks a hard time about going out and leaving her at home with a babysitter. If she knows her mom and dad have plans for the evening, she starts complaining of not feeling well that morning. After the babysitter arrives and her parents leave, Ashley keeps calling her mother on her cell phone, checking to make sure she's okay and asking "When are you coming home?" Ashley's terrified that something awful is going to happen to her mom and that she'll never see her again.

There's no doubt that Ashley has separation anxiety disorder. She's too old to be so frightened of being apart from her mom. By nine she should be able to sleep alone in her own bed and stay home with a babysitter without becoming distraught. Her worries about the safety of her mother, and her need to check on her with frequent cell phone calls, also are a concern and further confirm that this child has a problem with separation anxiety.

On the positive side, Ashley has no trouble going to school or other places where she'll be away from her mom and her home. She participates in numerous after-school and weekend activities (like gymnastics and Hebrew school), goes on lots of play dates, and has many close friends.

Kevin

Suddenly Kevin will not go to school. He had a problem separating from his mom when he began kindergarten, but that lasted only a couple of days. Now it's the middle of second grade and Kevin has missed weeks of school. Although he knows he sounds like a baby, he tells his mom, "I'm scared to go."

School is not the only place where Kevin is having problems. He's no longer able to go next door to play with his friend Antonio. If the two boys want to get together, it has to be at Kevin's house. He also has quit taking karate lessons. His dad used to take him to the classes, but now he doesn't want to be there without his mom.

Kevin also is having nightmares. He often dreams he's being kidnapped or that he's falling off a high cliff. He wakes up screaming, thinking he's in danger or that maybe he has died.

It's clear that Kevin has problems leaving home without his mother. He's not able to go to school, he can't go next door to see his friend, and he stopped karate—something he loved—all because he's anxious when he's not with his mom. Kevin also frequently has nightmares that have separation-related themes, a symptom that's particularly common in younger kids with separation anxiety disorder.

Unlike Ashley, Kevin has trouble leaving his mom and going away from home, but he's okay being at home when she's not there. For example, he's fine staying with a babysitter or being at home with Dad and his brothers. In fact he often has friends over at these times. He also can go places away from home as long as his mom is with him. But since that's not always possible (or the best way to handle things—something we'll discuss when we get into strategies for dealing with separation anxiety disorder), Kevin's missing out on a lot.

Cecelia

Cecelia is excited about starting middle school. But after the first few days she tells her mom she feels sick and doesn't want to go. A visit to the pediatrician shows there's nothing medically wrong with her. The doctor says it's probably just her "nerves" and that it will go away when she gets used to the new school. So her mom insists Cecelia go to school every day, but it's a battle each morning.

Looking back, Cecelia's mom admits her daughter had trouble adjusting to new situations in the past, always seeming to be "a step behind" most of her peers. She wasn't able to do a lot of the things other kids her age were able to, like going to sleepover parties, on overnight class trips, or to sleep-away camp. Whenever she had the choice, Cecelia seemed to prefer hanging out with her mom rather than socialize with her friends.

Cecelia's mom thought her daughter would become more independent when she got older, but instead she's taken a major step back, now having trouble going to school.

Cecelia probably had separation anxiety disorder long before she started middle school, but it wasn't until she had trouble going to school that her family realized she had a problem. The things she couldn't do during elementary school—mostly situations involving sleeping away from home—didn't seem like that big a deal, and her parents figured she'd grow out of it when she got older. They also thought she'd want to spend more time with friends—rather than her mother—as time went on. But rather than getting better, Cecelia's separation anxiety has gotten worse. She's having a very difficult time making the transition to middle school.

Cecelia *does*, however, go to school, so she's not missing out on the academic and social experiences that Kevin is. But she fights going almost every day, and this is making life at home with her family very tense.

Brandon

Brandon has a lot of worries for a five-year-old boy. Almost every day he's scared that something bad is going to happen to him—like he'll get kidnapped on the playground at recess or lost when he's at the mall with his mother. He worries a lot about his mom, too—that she'll be in an accident or get really sick and have to go to the hospital.

Brandon sticks very close to his mom even when they're at home. He always wants to be in the same room she's in. In fact, he even insists she leave the bathroom door open when she's taking a shower. Brandon still sleeps in his parents' bed even though he has a really great room of his own. He says he's just not ready to sleep alone yet.

Even though Brandon is only five, he already has separation anxiety disorder. His worries all are separation-related and too frequent to be considered normal. Although it's not unusual for kids this age to want to be close to their moms, Brandon should be able to handle being in a separate room (without having to have his mom leave the bathroom door open) and able to sleep in his own bed.

Brandon doesn't like being away from home, and away from his mom, unless it's really necessary. Fortunately, though, despite not wanting to be away from his mom, he *is* able to go to kindergarten. He also has friends, but because of his problem they usually come over to his house.

Separation Anxiety and School Refusal

As we discussed earlier, reluctance or refusal to go to school occurs in kids with separation anxiety disorder (as in Kevin and Cecelia's cases), but it's *not required* for the diagnosis. You may wonder, then, how common is it?

Facts about Separation Anxiety Disorder

Children with separation anxiety disorder tend to be *younger* than kids with other types of anxiety disorders.

Separation anxiety disorder is *more common in girls* than boys.

Many children with separation anxiety live in *single-parent households*.

The disorder usually has a *shorter duration* than the other childhood anxiety disorders.

The disorder is *episodic*, not chronic.

Some kids have only one episode, but others have multiple episodes with symptom-free periods between them.

Specific phobia and *generalized anxiety disorder* are the only other anxiety disorders typically seen in children with separation anxiety disorder.

Apparently it's quite common, at least among children seen in mental health settings. In fact, data collected in the 1980s at our Pittsburgh clinic and published in the *American Journal of Psychiatry* showed that almost three-quarters of children with separation anxiety disorder have trouble going to school. (Since a child's refusal to go to school often is the trigger that drives parents to seek professional help, it may be that kids with separation anxiety who aren't seen in mental health settings are less likely to have this problem.)

> **The majority of kids who receive treatment for separation anxiety disorder have anxiety about going to school.**

Although children with separation anxiety disorder often avoid a lot of situations, not going to school undoubtedly has the most serious consequences. Substantial time away from school interferes with many aspects of a child's development. It interferes with learning and academic achievement, the development of social skills and formation of peer relationships, and the acquisition of important "self-control" skills, like the ability to control impulses, delay gratification, and sustain attention. Staying at home, rather than going out into the world—to school— also hampers kids from developing feelings of independence and autonomy and can adversely affect their self-esteem. It's hard for kids to feel good about themselves when they aren't able to do what's expected of them.

You should be aware that anxiety about going to school, as part of separation anxiety disorder, often first develops following a prolonged absence from school—like after Christmas or spring break, summer vacation, or following a lengthy illness that requires a child to stay home. Kids get used to being at home and close to their parents and then have difficulty parting when the vacation or illness is over.

You probably have heard the term *school phobia* before and may be curious about how this differs from the school refusal seen in separation anxiety disorder. Although the end result, as far as school is concerned, is pretty much the same, there are some important differences between these two types of kids.

Children with school phobia are afraid of going to school because of some aspect of the school environment. For example, a child like this may be scared of a bully at school, afraid of a teacher, embarrassed about getting undressed in front of other kids in gym, or anxious giving book reports in front of the class. (We'll talk about this in greater depth in Chapters 7 and 8, when we get to social and specific phobias.) On the other hand, children with separation anxiety disorder are afraid to go to school because they are nervous about being away from their moms or their homes (or both).

Children with separation anxiety who are afraid to go to school may be willing to go if a parent goes along with them. For example, Li, a first grader, convinced his mom to stay in her car in the school parking lot *for the whole school day* so that he would be able to go. (You'd be surprised by how many parents are willing to do this, thinking it's going to help their kids. While doing this can be a useful *step* in getting a child with separation anxiety back to school, as you'll see later on when we talk about strategies to overcome this problem, it's not a long-term solution.)

Kids with separation anxiety disorder who don't go to school (either because a parent won't accompany them or because they're anxious about just being away from home) almost always want to be at home. This differs from kids with phobias who are afraid to go to school. Phobic children don't necessarily want to be at home; they just don't want to be at school (or to confront the particular aspect of the school environment that causes their anxiety).

An especially scary feature of school refusal for parents is when a child threatens "I'll kill myself if you make me go!" When children with separation anxiety disorder threaten suicide or, even worse, make gestures like they're going to hurt themselves, they almost always don't really want to be dead. They're trying to—in the strongest sense of the word—persuade their parents to let them stay home. As you can imagine, this approach usually is very effective. (However, if your child is threatening suicide, *please do not take it upon yourself* to figure out if he or she is serious or just trying to manipulate you. Take your child to a professional for an evaluation and let the doctor determine what's going on and how it should be handled.)

In trying to get out of going to school, kids sometimes take other types of drastic measures—other than threatening to, or making gestures about, committing "suicide"—and can end up accidentally injuring themselves. I've heard from a number of parents of kids who have tried to get out of cars (sometimes while they were moving!) on the way to school. Elementary school teachers have told me about children with separation anxiety jumping out of classroom windows (thankfully, always on the ground or first floor) so they can get away from school and go home. Before you become alarmed, please keep in mind that, although behavior like this does occur, it's rare and happens in only the most severe of cases.

Children with separation anxiety disorder who won't go to school—and even some who don't have a problem with school—may be perceived of as "controlling" by their families. For example, Max's mom says, "It's like *he's* in charge of our family." This shift in power usually occurs because parents are frightened by, and don't know how to deal with, the out-of-control behavior (tantrums, threats, hysterics) they see in their kids. Consequently they respond by acquiescing to their children's demands.

While it's very easy to understand why parents behave this way, letting children avoid separation situations actually ends up *making them worse* (*more* separation anxious). We'll talk about better ways for you to deal with your child's avoidance behavior later in the chapter.

The Episodic Nature of Separation Anxiety Disorder

As I mentioned in the sidebar on page 90, separation anxiety disorder occurs in episodes. By "episodes," I mean that the disorder takes place during one or more distinct periods (of varying lengths), each with a beginning and an end. (As you'll see when we get to some of the other childhood anxiety disorders, not all of them are episodic—some are, instead, chronic.) While many kids have only one episode of separation anxiety disorder, other children have two, three, or even more.

The duration of an episode can range from a month to years. And the length of time between episodes also varies—it can be weeks, months, or years from one episode to the next.

Wendy had her first episode of separation anxiety disorder when she started kindergarten. It lasted about three months, and then she was fine—until the third grade, when her family moved and she had to change schools. This time the problem went on longer, all the way through the fourth grade. Although she then recovered, at the beginning of middle school Wendy's separation anxiety returned once more. By eleven she had had three episodes of the disorder.

Trevor, who now is in high school, was more fortunate than Wendy. He had a brief episode of separation anxiety disorder when he was eight and never had another.

Who is at risk for having an episode of separation anxiety disorder? First, children who have had a previous episode (or episodes) have a greater chance of having additional ones. Second, kids who have a history of subclinical separation anxiety (they don't meet all of the criteria for the disorder but definitely show signs of the problem) may go on to develop an episode. Finally, children with anxious temperaments or those who have family members with anxiety disorders are at a somewhat greater risk.

Life Events That Can Trigger an Episode

Children who are at risk for separation anxiety disorder are particularly vulnerable at certain times in their lives. Life experiences (including the ones we just discussed for Wendy) that often are associated with the onset of episodes are listed on the facing page. As you look at the situations on the list you'll notice that a number of them are normal developmental transitions that all kids go through. Although common, these times of change can be especially tough for the kids who are the subject of this chapter.

Knowing which events or circumstances may bring on an episode of separation anxiety disorder allows you to make preparations or take actions that possibly will circumvent a potential problem. While there's no guarantee of success, there's no question that with separation anxiety disorder forewarned is forearmed.

You'll also notice that many of the life events in the sidebar were already discussed in Chapter 3. While I won't go into them in detail again now (you can refer back to the last chapter), I want to reemphasize certain important points and also talk about experiences that weren't already covered.

Events That Can Trigger an Episode
of Separation Anxiety Disorder

First "school-like" experience (nursery school, preschool)

Beginning kindergarten or first grade

Starting middle school or junior high

Being out of school at home for a week or more (vacation, illness, death in family)

Separation from parent or home for a week or more

Illness or death of a close relative, family friend, or peer

Move to a new home

Change of schools

Onset of puberty

The transition from elementary school to middle school (or to junior high, depending on which state your child lives in) is a time when many kids develop episodes of separation anxiety disorder. Several factors can make this transition even more difficult and further increase the likelihood that your child will have a problem. For one thing, the younger (chronologically) or more immature (emotionally) your child is, the greater the chance he or she will have trouble adjusting. Also important is how different the new school is from your child's old school. Is the new school building *much larger*? Are there *many* more students there? Is it in another part of town, one your child isn't familiar with? Are your child's friends going to the same school or a different one?

Entering puberty is another time when kids can have problems with separation anxiety, particularly for girls who begin menstruating somewhat early (around ten or eleven), while they're still in elementary school. These kids sometimes take a "step back" developmentally and have trouble separating because they're anxious about becoming adolescents and, ultimately, adults.

Although I discussed this earlier when we talked about separation anxiety and school refusal, it can't be stated enough how often kids develop problems with separation after being out of school at home for an extended period of time. Even if your child has no trouble going back to school, you may find that he or she wants to stick closer to you or to home after a school vacation or a lengthy illness that required a stay at home.

Physical loss of or separation from a parent (because of a premature death, marital separation or divorce, a hospitalization, lengthy business travel) or a child's being away from home for a prolonged period of time (attending boarding school; going to sleep-away camp) also can trigger an episode of separation anxiety disorder.

Stopping an Episode before It Starts

There are many things you can do to help ward off a potential episode of separation anxiety disorder. Obviously stopping an episode before it starts is better than having to deal with one that's already in progress.

My suggestions have been written for parents, but you may find it beneficial to share some of the information included here with other adults (teachers, camp counselors, grandparents) who play important roles in your child's life.

1. Familiarize your child with the separation situation before it happens.

Unfamiliar circumstances—places, people, and events—are more likely to generate anxiety than those that are familiar. Your child will be less likely to become overly anxious when faced with a separation situation if you familiarize him or her, as much as possible, with different aspects of the situation *before* the separation actually is to take place.

For example, five-year-old Allie's parents are going to leave her with a new babysitter this weekend. Her mom arranged for the babysitter to come over during the week so Allie could get acquainted with her. The three of them—Allie, her mom, and the babysitter—talked, played games, and had snacks. When the weekend came and it was time to leave Allie alone with the babysitter, Allie's mom could see that her daughter felt comfortable and relaxed. The separation situation was not entirely novel—Allie had already been exposed to many aspects of it.

Another common separation situation that can cause a lot of anxiety is when children are beginning or changing schools. To help make this easier for her child, Barry's mom took him to the school to meet his teacher and become familiar with the physical environment of the school (the room that will be his classroom; the layout of the building) before school started. If your son or daughter is just beginning school, it's also a good idea for your child to get to know some of the other kids who will be in the same class before the beginning of the school year. Since children who will be entering the same kindergarten or first-grade class usually live in the same neighborhood, arranging this shouldn't be too difficult. You may want to consider having a "before school starts" party (goodies to eat and games to play) so the kids can get together and get to know each other in a pleasant, nonstressful setting. (If your child will be entering a school where admission is not based on geographical location, the school may be willing to arrange introductions between you and your child and other sets of parents and children before the start of the school year.)

2. Start with small separations first and then proceed in a "stepwise" manner.

Children at risk for separation anxiety may develop an episode when a separation situation that is "too big" is attempted prematurely. For example, Abbey's parents made plans for her to go to sleep-away camp for two weeks even though she was still having problems staying overnight at friends' homes. Because she wasn't ready to be away from home that long, the camp experience ended up being "a disaster." Abbey had to leave before the two weeks were up.

When parents are trying to get their children comfortable in situations where they will be away from them or from home, it's best to start with easier situations first—those that cause very little anxiety—and then, once these are "mastered," move on to progressively more difficult ones. In Abbey's case her parents probably should have increased the frequency of her overnights so that she became more comfortable with them before attempting something more difficult. They then could have tried having her sleep away from home two or three nights (maybe at a relative's home who lives close by) as an "intermediate" step before progressing to longer stays away from home.

You can determine the approximate difficulty of a particular situation by keeping in mind that separation anxiety is very much influenced by the duration of the separation experience and the physical proximity of your child to you and/or home. Shorter periods of time and shorter distances almost always produce less anxiety than longer time periods and larger distances.

Once your child becomes comfortable with a particular separation situation, the situation can be made harder by incrementally increasing the duration and/or distance. This should be done using your child's own reactions as a guide to what pace to follow.

> **The level of anxiety you can expect often depends on the duration of the separation and the distance your child will be from you or home.**

Five-year-old Kristy is fine playing at the next-door neighbor's house, but she won't go on play dates any farther away from home than that. As a first step she and her mom agreed she would try to go to Amanda's, who lives across the street and three doors down, for a half hour. Once she was okay with this Kristy agreed to stay at Amanda's for a longer period of time—for an hour. As she became comfortable spending increasingly longer periods at Amanda's home, Kristy's mom suggested that her daughter try a half hour at Tia's house, which is farther away from their home (two blocks away). Kristy and her mom continued to work on her play dates being farther and farther away from home and for progressively longer periods of time.

One separation situation that all children ultimately must face is going to school for the first time. While it's often helpful to get children to start to attend school by going with them (to the school building or into the classroom) for the first few days, parents should fade themselves out of the school environment as soon as possible.

Also, it's not a good idea to visit your child during the school day (at recess on the playground; in the cafeteria at lunchtime) or take a volunteer or paid position at your child's school because your physical proximity is likely to *increase* your child's separation anxiety (even though it may decrease *yours*).

Sometimes parents have difficulty determining what independent behaviors ("separation steps") are appropriate for a child at a certain age (this frequently is the case if it's a family's first child). Angelica's parents aren't sure at what age she should be able to sleep overnight at a friend's home without a problem. Bridget's mom and dad wonder when it's reasonable to expect their daughter to be able to be home alone during the day for short periods of time.

Ultimately each family must come up with their own decisions regarding these issues. When in doubt, though, it can be helpful to speak with other parents who already have been through this with their own children or to consult professionals who specialize in fields that focus on children's behavior (teachers, pediatricians, child psychologists) to get their read on the topic.

3. Use "transitional objects" during separations.

When children are going to be away from their parents and home, it's a good idea to send them off with one or more items—things that remind them of their family or home or other things they're attached to—to help them be more at ease. Using "transitional objects," as they often are referred to, decreases separation anxiety and assists your child in moving on to more autonomous and independent behavior.

Whenever Monica spends a night away from home—at her grandparents' or a friend's house—she takes along her

> Transitional objects— things that remind your child of you or home— can help reduce anxiety during separations.

blanket, her nightlight, and her favorite stuffed animal so she feels more at home. On the first day of school Charlotte felt comforted by the picture of her dog her mom put in her lunch box. When Eden was leaving for his overnight class trip, he asked his dad if he could take one of his ties to keep with him while he was away.

There are some kids, however, who become *more* anxious during separations when they keep with them things that clearly remind them of family members. Take Lani for example. Rather than helping her, the family photo she took with her to camp made her cry every time she looked at it. For children like Lani it's better to use objects from home that they are attached to (a special toy, pillow, etc.), rather than things that are more directly related to the person they will miss. (Unfortunately the only way to find out what works best for your child is by trial and error. On the positive side, though, it usually takes just one separation experience to find out if something intended to help is hindering instead.)

4. Use rewards to reinforce the behavior you want.

When children are successful at separating, it is very important to reward them for their efforts. Reinforcement can take the form of verbal praise, a material possession, or a special situation or event (going to an amusement park; seeing a new movie).

Praise works well with almost all children. But if you're going to use a material reward or an event, make sure it's something your child really wants or else it won't be effective. It's also worth pointing out that material rewards don't necessarily have to cost much. As you know, kids—especially when they're younger—can get very excited about things that cost very little. And some events that can work as rewards don't cost anything.

To be most effective reinforcement should take place shortly, in fact as soon as possible, after the separation has occurred. Praise, of course, always can be administered on the spot. When it's not feasible to give a reward immediately, as often is the case with rewards that are activities, tokens can serve in the short run as "intermediaries" for the reward. Your child can then turn them in to you later, just before receiving the reward.

Tokens really can be almost anything. Some of the more popular choices include plastic chips (from game sets), metallic stars, or stickers. Have your child pick the one he or she likes best. That way you'll be sure it has the most impact.

5. Discourage avoidance and escape behavior.

If you've followed suggestions 1 through 4, it's less likely your child will try to avoid or escape from (basically run out of) separation situations. However, if this should occur, you should encourage your child to try to face or "stick out" the situation. Avoiding or escaping it will *increase* your child's separation anxiety—your child will be more likely to react similarly (avoid or escape the same situation) when confronted with it again. (This occurs via *negative* reinforcement, where the termination of something aversive serves as a "reward" for behavior and, consequently, increases the likelihood that it will recur.)

There is, however, one exception to this rule. If your child truly is *not* ready for a certain separation experience—if it's too much of a "leap"—forcing the issue may very well make things worse. (This happens through the process of "sensitization," which I'll discuss a little later on.)

Even though she had trouble going to day camp last year, this summer Emma's parents decided to send her to sleep-away camp. They were hopeful she would do okay since she was now more mature and had been able to spend longer periods away from home successfully during the past school year.

Emma tried to get out of going, but her parents wouldn't hear of it. After she was gone just a couple of days her folks received a call from the camp's director telling them they had to come pick Emma up. He said she had "gone berserk" (in reality she was having panic attacks, but the camp director wasn't familiar with this type of anxiety reaction) and the camp was not equipped to deal with this kind of behavior.

After her ordeal at camp Emma was not the same child. Her separation anxiety was much worse and she couldn't do many of the things she previously was able to.

Although they had the best of intentions, Emma's parents exacerbated their daughter's separation anxiety by pushing her into a situation she wasn't ready for. In retrospect they probably should have tried day camp again, since Emma had had problems with that separation experience the summer before. After being successful with day camp, they then could have moved on to an intermediate step—something more difficult than day camp but not as hard as an entire summer at sleep-away camp. Ultimately, with effort and time, Emma eventually would have been able to go to sleep-away camp.

While I want to caution you about what can happen in a situation like Emma's, please don't let this child's experience deter you from encouraging your child to participate in increasingly challenging separation situations. It's just that you need to be careful that you don't "overshoot the mark" and unintentionally make things worse rather than better. If you're not sure whether your child is ready for a particular separation experience, it never hurts to get an opinion from an expert. While it might cost a bit now, the grief it will save you later will be well worth it.

While we're on the subject of summer camp, many parents have asked me what to do if their child begs to come home on "parents' day," usually held in the middle of the camp season. In some cases children simply aren't ready to spend that long a period of time away from home. But for many other kids the distress they show during their parents' visit disappears almost instantly once their folks have left.

Clearly the decision of whether to make a child stay on when he or she is distraught is a difficult one. It's important to weigh the potential negative effects of letting your child leave a separation situation prematurely (and reinforcing escape behavior) versus the possibility of your child continuing to be distressed and possibly feeling abandoned during the remaining weeks of camp. The only real guidance I can give you here is to think about similar experiences your child has had in the past. Does your child usually get over separation distress once you're out of the picture? If the answer is "yes," your child probably will be fine once you've gone home.

Ending an Episode Once It's Begun

If you're reading this chapter while your child is having a separation anxiety episode, the guidelines for prevention obviously aren't going to work for you. In this case the steps you need to take to help your child are techniques that mental health professionals use successfully to treat this problem.

Unfortunately, as I said at the beginning of this chapter, separation anxiety disorder usually does not get better on its own. Actually research suggests that if you do not attend to the problem, your child is likely to get worse (have an episode become more severe or have additional episodes) as time goes on. The good news, though, is that with the appropriate intervention almost all children with this disorder get better and do so pretty quickly.

You may be saying to yourself, "How will I be able to do what a trained professional can do for my child?" While certainly no parent can be expected to have the skills of someone who specializes in this area, most of the treatment methods that have been proven to work for separation anxiety disorder *can be learned* by moms and dads.

Parents are especially likely to be successful on their own (without professional help) if it's early on in their child's episode and the separation anxiety is on the mild to moderate side. However, if the problem already has gone on for a long time and/or your child's separation anxiety is very severe (for example, he or she has missed months of school), or you just don't feel comfortable handling it on your own, seek professional help.

1. Identify the problem and start your intervention as early in the episode as possible.

Identifying an episode early on and taking the correct actions will shorten its duration and, consequently, the negative effects the disorder has on your child and your family.

As you'll recall from our discussion earlier, the criteria for diagnosing separation anxiety disorder specify that a child must have the problem for at least four weeks. However, for parents there is no benefit to waiting this long to start to deal with the problem.

If your child has at least three of the symptoms listed on page 83 for separation anxiety disorder, in my opinion it's time to intervene even if it hasn't gone on for a month. The goal here is to nip the episode in the bud, not to wait till it's gone on long enough to qualify for a formal psychiatric diagnosis.

Mary has been at home with the flu for two weeks. She now seems to be over the illness (her fever and most of the other symptoms are gone), and the pediatrician has given the go-ahead for her to return to school. Despite her apparent medical recovery, Mary continues to complain of physical symptoms—"feels achy all over"—and says she can't go back to school. After a few days of this Mary's mom became suspicious and asked her child about what was really going on. Mary finally admitted she's very nervous about going back to school. She has a feeling that something bad will happen to her if she leaves her mom and her home.

Now that Mary's mom knows her child is having trouble with separation anxiety, she can address the real problem. However, consider what might have happened if she had accepted Mary's statement that she wasn't entirely well and let her continue to stay out of school. Mary might have had *an additional* couple of weeks at home before the reason behind her school avoidance became clear. If this occurred, the extra time away from school would have made separating from her mother to go back to school even more difficult.

That's because, in most cases, the longer a separation situation is avoided, the more difficult it is for a child to overcome the fear.

> **The longer a separation situation is avoided, the more difficult it will be for your child to overcome the fear.**

Remember the old saying "If you fall off a horse, get right back on it again"? The same principle applies to separation anxiety disorder. The sooner you can get your child back into the situation that's being avoided, the better off he or she will be.

2. Educate your child about separation anxiety.

Research studies, including ones conducted by our own group reported in 1998 in the *Journal of the American Academy of Child and Adolescent Psychiatry*, have shown the value of educational materials in treating separation anxiety disorder. Often referred to as "bibliotherapy," this treatment technique involves providing written information to children so they'll get a better understanding of their problem. Usually these materials include suggestions for how to approach separation anxiety by using examples of other (fictional) kids and how they successfully faced and overcame their fears. In addition to educating children, this approach helps kids by letting them know they're not alone—that other children experience similar problems.

For young children the simplest, most effective way of providing this information is by having your child read a book (or reading it to him or her) that focuses on the issue of separation anxiety. There are a number of good ones that have been written for kids ages five through eight, including *The Runaway Bunny* and *The Good-Bye Book*. For older children, and for some younger kids who are more sophisticated, parents can share much of the information in this chapter.

3. Create a fear list and have your child confront the fears.

The really essential ingredient to getting rid of separation anxiety is having children confront the situations they fear. While this may seem like common sense, it's the particular *way* that kids tackle their fears that determines whether they'll be successful or not.

The method that's used is called *graduated exposure.* It's similar to the stepwise approach we touched on earlier when we talked about prevention. Kids start by facing situations that cause low levels of anxiety and then gradually move on to increasingly difficult situations, that is, ones that cause more anxiety.

Constructing a list of the separation situations your child fears will give you and your child the steps to use for exposure as well as the order in which to approach them. The list should contain ten items that describe, as specifically as possible, separation situations your child frequently encounters that cause varying degrees of anxiety. Items 1 and 2, then, should be situations that trigger minimal anxiety. The items that come next should be increasingly difficult, with the final item—10—being the most difficult, or anxiety producing, of them all.

I suggest you come up with the items by creating them together with your child. But if your child is unable or unwilling to work with you on this, you can generate them on your own. Here are three items that Francine's mom came up with for her five-year-old daughter:

Item 1   Fifteen minutes alone in your room while Mom is in the kitchen

Item 2   A one-hour play date at Maribel's house (next door)

Item 3   Sleep in your bedroom for a whole night

To help make sure you're on the right track with how you arrange the items on your child's list, keep in mind that as anxiety increases the likelihood of escape or avoidance behavior also increases. So if your child repeatedly refuses to do something or always leaves a situation early (because of separation anxiety), that situation probably should be one of the higher items on the list.

You and your child can use a numerical scale to assign fear scores to the items so it's clear exactly where to place them on the list. For young children (five or six years old) a very simple scale, like this one, usually works best: 0 = not nervous or scared at all ("no problem"); 1 = a little nervous or scared ("a little problem"); 2 = very nervous or scared ("a big problem").

For older kids (or younger kids who are able to do this) a scale with more gradations can be used, like the one on the facing page, which takes into consideration avoidance behavior as well as fear level. Again, if your child doesn't want to participate in this, you can rate the items yourself. With the fear scores to guide you, put your child's final fear list on the form on page 108.

Now that you've made the list, your child can start working on approaching the separation situations beginning with item 1 (the easiest one). Arrange for your child to have as many opportunities as possible to be in this situation. By doing it over and over again, your child eventually will get used to the situation and it no longer will cause anxiety. Once this happens you can move on to the next item on the list, but *do not go on to a more difficult situation until your child is comfortable in the one you currently are working on.* One by one, using the same approach, have your child tackle each of the items until the final item on the list is completed.

I can't say how many exposures it will take your child to be okay in a particular situation, but it's safe to assume that the higher

Fear Scale

0   Doesn't avoid the situation; isn't nervous or scared at all

1   Hesitates to enter the situation but rarely avoids it; is a little nervous or scared

2   Sometimes avoids the situation; definitely nervous or scared

3   Usually avoids the situation; very nervous or scared

4   Always avoids the situation; nervous or scared to the point of panic

items on the list (the ones that produce the most anxiety) will take more times. To get the most out of the exposures it's best to have them occur close together—one or more times a week or even, if possible, daily—rather than having lengthy periods of time between them. Of course it won't be feasible for children to be in certain separation situations as frequently as others (for example, sleeping overnight at the same friend's house several times a week probably won't be possible, unless your child's friend has unusually helpful parents). You should know, though, that the less frequent the exposure, the more difficult it will be for your child's anxiety to subside. (In fact, if a separation situation triggers extremely high anxiety, having your child confront it infrequently actually can be worse than not having him or her confront it at all. The exposure can increase rather than decrease your child's anxiety through the process of "sensitization," which I mentioned briefly earlier. The anxiety in that one situation then can spread or "generalize" to other separation situations so that your child backslides and can't do things he or she used to. You may remember this was the case for Emma, discussed earlier.)

Having your child face separation situations one step at a time is an integral part of getting past separation anxiety disorder. By carefully constructing a list of fears and repeatedly confronting each one, your child will be well on the way to overcoming this problem.

Your Child's Fear List

Item 1 (the easiest situation)

_____

Item 2

_____

Item 3

_____

Item 4

_____

Item 5

_____

Item 6

_____

Item 7

_____

Item 8

_____

Item 9

_____

Item 10 (the hardest situation)

_____

4. Help your child develop and use coping skills when anticipating and facing separation situations.

There are several techniques, often referred to as *coping skills*, that can help your child in separation situations. These methods are good for reducing anxiety when your child is anticipating a separation or actually confronting one. Encourage your child to use them when tackling the situations on his or her fear list.

Positive Thoughts

In Chapter 1 we talked about how anxiety often includes upsetting or catastrophic thoughts. For kids with separation anxiety disorder these thoughts frequently focus on something terrible happening to them or their parents.

These thoughts often are considered a byproduct of anxiety, but they also end up increasing kids' fear levels. For that reason it's very helpful to teach kids how to replace these types of thoughts with more positive and helpful ones that will decrease their anxiety and help them cope better with separations.

The first step in using this technique is for your child to learn to recognize anxiety-producing thoughts as they occur. If your child tends to share his or her private upsetting thoughts with you or verbalizes them out loud, you can help by pointing out when this is happening. Your child also can work on this when you aren't around by paying attention to when he or she is feeling anxious and then "backtracking" to the thoughts. Another way to get at the thoughts is by having children close their eyes and asking them to imagine they're in a separation situation that causes them anxiety (it's best if it's one that's happened recently) and then asking them what they're thinking.

Once the anxiety-producing thoughts have been identified, the next step is for you and your child to come up with alternative positive thoughts that can be used to replace or counter the negative thoughts.

Desiree told her mom that she sometimes thinks, "I'm going to be kidnapped" when she's on the playground at recess. Together Desiree and her mom decided it might be a good idea to come back at this thought by saying "The other kids and my teacher are here. Nothing bad is going to happen." (The specific thoughts that will be effective are different for different children, so I can't give you the ones to use with your child. As for Desiree and her mom, you and your child will need to come up with these together.)

Kids can say their new positive thoughts silently in their heads or, if they are by themselves, they can say them out loud. The important thing is that they *do* say them whenever they are having the upsetting thoughts. This, of course, will take practice.

Susie, age eight, gets very anxious when she's waiting after school for her mother to pick her up. If her mom is even a couple of minutes late, she thinks, "She's been in a car accident" and "I'll never see her again." With practice Susie was able to replace these thoughts with "Mom probably ran into traffic" and "My mom always shows up." Using these substitute thoughts helped Susie decrease her anxiety, and she was more comfortable waiting for her mother to arrive.

Pleasant Imagery

Pleasant imagery is another helpful technique for kids with separation anxiety disorder. Basically it involves having children close their eyes and conjure up a (predetermined) pleasant mental image of a happy place or time from their past.

Children should choose their pleasant images themselves. Kids often pick special places that bring them comfort. For example, Carlos decided to use the backyard at his grandma's house as his pleasant image. Melanie chose her family's summer cabin. Some kids use interactions with family members or their pets instead of places.

Once they've selected their scene children should use it whenever they're feeling anxious. It's easiest for kids to use pleasant imagery when they're by themselves in a relatively quiet place. When this isn't possible, accommodations usually can be made so the technique still can be utilized successfully.

During an overnight stay at her friend's house ten-year-old Donna was feeling very anxious. Early in the evening she thought about calling her mom and asking to come home but decided to try using the pleasant imagery technique instead. She told her friend she needed to use the bathroom. Alone there Donna was able to conjure up her pleasant scene. It worked and she was feeling much better until after "lights out," when the anxiety came back and she couldn't fall asleep. Since she was lying in bed with her eyes closed anyway, it was easy for her to use the imagery technique again. Once more it worked, and she was soon asleep.

Some kids are better at using imagery than others. If you think your child may have a problem with this, it's a good idea to have him or her practice coming up with the pleasant scene in a non-anxiety-producing environment before attempting to use it during a separation. If your child just doesn't seem to have the ability to produce mental pictures or images, pass on this technique and use the other methods described in this section.

Deep Breathing

Deep breathing—breathing slowly and deeply from the diaphragm—is a relaxation method that counteracts anxiety. It's particularly good for kids who tend to hyperventilate (breathe shallowly and rapidly) when they're frightened.

The technique involves taking a deep breath through the nose (never the mouth!) very slowly, to a count of three ("breathe in, two, three"), then slowly exhaling, again through the nose and to the count of three ("relax [*exhale*], two, three"). Your child must take the breath from deep down within the abdomen ("the lower stomach," as kids sometimes call it), not from the upper portion of the chest, for this technique to be effective.

If this is done correctly, your child's abdomen actually should extend somewhat. (I sometimes ask kids to place one hand on their "lower stomach" so they can feel it moving outward.) Another way to make sure that children are doing the breathing exercise correctly is to watch that their shoulders do not rise upward (a sure sign that breathing is taking place from the upper chest and not from the abdomen).

Children should first learn and practice this technique with their eyes closed in a relaxed place, like their bedrooms, perhaps before going to sleep (assuming that sleeping alone isn't a situation that triggers separation anxiety). Ten repetitions (each inhale–exhale combination counts as one repetition) once a day for a couple of weeks usually is enough time for kids to get the hang of it.

Once your child is able to use the technique comfortably in a nonthreatening situation it can be used when he or she is anxious. The great thing about this relaxation method is that once kids are good at doing it they don't need to be alone (or have their eyes shut) to utilize it. Other kids won't even know they're using it.

5. Create a reward program to reinforce your child's accomplishments.

As we discussed earlier, material objects and special events (and your praise too!) can be used to reinforce your child's new behavior.

Together with your child, come up with two lists of rewards. The first list should consist of small rewards that will be used each time a separation situation on the fear list is confronted. The second list should contain larger rewards you'll give after your child has advanced to a new (harder) item on the fear list.

Eight-year-old Morgan and his mom decided to use movie rentals and Morgan's favorite foods as small rewards. On his list of large rewards they included going go-cart racing, playing video games at the arcade at the mall, and going to Chuck E. Cheese's for dinner. Leah, age eleven, had an assortment of grooming products (lip gloss; a new kind of hair gel) as her small rewards and a list of CDs she wanted as her large rewards.

In addition to using objects and events as rewards, it can be helpful (especially for young kids) to use a calendarlike chart where you place a sticker (or star or checkmark, depending on your child's preference) on each day your child confronts one of his or her fears. The chart should be hung in a place where your child will frequently see it—like on the refrigerator door or in your daughter or son's bedroom. Seeing the days and weeks fill up with stickers gives kids another confirmation of their achievements.

The calendar also can serve as an intermediary step toward obtaining a particular reward. For instance, you and your child can agree that a certain number of stickers in a week (or a month) will earn a really big reward, like going on an overnight trip with the family or getting a special toy or game he or she has been wanting for a long time.

As you've seen in this chapter, the heart of dealing with separation anxiety disorder is to have kids face the situations they fear. Together with coping skills to decrease anxiety and a reward program to reinforce new behavior, you now have all the tools you need to help your child overcome this anxiety problem.

5 "BUT MOM, WHAT IF ... ?!"
Generalized Anxiety Disorder

Nine-year-old Lynn is a "worry wart." She's preoccupied with how she's doing in school even though she always gets straight A's. An excellent athlete, Lynn is the goalie for the neighborhood soccer team. But despite her success, she gets really anxious before each game because she's worried about how she's going to play.

Lynn often has trouble falling asleep at night because of upsetting thoughts that keep going around in her head. She also gets stomachaches two or three times a week that the doctor says are caused by stress.

Lynn's parents try to reassure her that everything will be okay, but rather than benefiting, she seems to be getting worse. What should Lynn's folks do? How can they help their daughter get control of her worries?

Children begin developing the ability to anticipate the future between the ages of two and four. By the time they're in elementary school they're able to come up with a variety of possible outcomes for many different types of situations.

The ability to anticipate a negative outcome serves many important functions, not the least of which is to help protect kids from danger. Some children, though, become so overly concerned and preoccupied with the possibility of bad things happening that the adaptive or helpful aspect of negative anticipation is lost. This is the case for children who have generalized anxiety disorder.

Worrying is the hallmark of generalized anxiety disorder. Although normal children, as discussed in Chapter 1, also have worries, the worries of generalized anxiety disorder are different. They are more intense, more frequent, more varied, and experienced as uncontrollable. They cause a great deal of distress and interfere with different aspects of your child's life.

Unlike separation anxiety disorder, the focus of the last chapter, generalized anxiety disorder tends to be a chronic condition. Usually it starts during childhood and—if unattended to—continues into adolescence and then adulthood, often lasting a lifetime.

Your child's future does not have to follow this course! Identifying the problem early on—that is, *now*—and doing something about it can make a tremendous difference in how things turn out for your child. That's because generalized anxiety disorder is a problem that's definitely best "nipped in the bud." The earlier you address it, the more likely you are to be successful. And the longer it continues, the more difficult it is to change.

In this chapter are the tools your child will need to overcome this anxiety disorder. But if you're to help your child use them optimally, it will be helpful to understand the disorder in depth. To start with, you should be aware that diagnosing generalized anxiety disorder can sometimes be a bit tricky.

Diagnosing Generalized Anxiety Disorder

The criteria used to diagnose generalized anxiety disorder in children have changed over the years, more so than for any of the other childhood anxiety disorders. Unfortunately, the changes have not reflected consensus among professionals in the field, and still to this day there is disagreement among experts about how best to define and diagnose this disorder in kids.

Because of this, and because how generalized anxiety disorder is defined affects whether your child will be viewed as having this problem, it's important for you to be aware of the different ways it has been (and currently is) conceptualized. Having the whole picture will put you in a better position to assess your son or daughter's situation, whether on your own or with the help of a mental health professional.

In 1968 the American Psychiatric Association created the diagnostic category "overanxious reaction" for children and adolescents who had excessive worries and other psychological and physical signs of anxiety. In the 1980s overanxious *reaction* was renamed overanxious *disorder*, but the essential features of the condition stayed pretty much the same.

The symptoms that a child must have to be diagnosed with overanxious disorder are listed in the sidebar below. Of the seven symptoms, five deal with some aspect of worrying: worrying about the future, worrying about the past, worrying about competence, worrying about how one is perceived, and the need for reassurance about worries. The remaining two focus on physical signs of anxiety: physical, or *somatic*, complaints (like stomachaches or headaches) and feeling tense or unable to relax. To receive a diagnosis of overanxious disorder kids have to experience at least four of the seven symptoms frequently for at least six months. However, the four (or more) symptoms *can not* be related exclusively to *another* anxiety disorder. Let me give you a couple of examples to help explain what I mean by this.

Symptoms of Overanxious Disorder

The child must have at least four of the following symptoms to receive this diagnosis. For six months or longer, the child frequently shows these signs of anxiety or worry:

- Is overly or unreasonably worried about upcoming events.
- Is overly or unreasonably concerned about past behavior.
- Is overly or unreasonably concerned about how well he or she is doing in one or more areas—sports, school, friendships, etc.
- Has stomach pains, headaches, or other physical complaints that don't have a medical explanation.
- Is extremely self-conscious.
- Needs an unusual level of reassurance about a number of things from parents, teachers, and other adults.
- Feels very tense or has great difficulty relaxing.

Ten-year-old Mikayla has four of the symptoms of overanxious disorder. Closer examination of each of her symptoms, though, shows they're actually part of a social phobia. Her worries about the future and the past are only about social situations. Her self-consciousness also is related to her social anxiety, and the stomachaches she frequently has occur just in anticipation of social events. Tommy, age eight, also has four symptoms. For him the symptoms are linked to his separation anxiety disorder.

Because the symptoms of both of these kids are related exclusively to other anxiety disorders, neither received the diagnosis of overanxious disorder. Eleven-year-old Burt, on the other hand, really does have overanxious disorder. His worries and other anxiety symptoms don't revolve around a single theme—they're related to many different things.

Although for more than twenty-five years there was a diagnosis specifically for overanxious children, when the fourth edition of DSM was published in 1994 (DSM-IV), this childhood anxiety disorder no longer was included. "Generalized anxiety disorder," or GAD, a diagnosis originally developed for and previously applied only to adults, now was to be used in its place.

Many mental health professionals who specialize in the diagnosis and treatment of children took issue with this change. One concern raised was whether an anxiety disorder diagnosis that had been created for adults really would be applicable to children, since children experience anxiety somewhat differently than adults.

The diagnosis of psychopathology in children has lagged considerably behind adult psychiatry. In fact, it's only within the last half century that the presence of psychiatric illness in children has been fully recognized (prior to this time, it was thought that children did not experience anxiety or depression, for example). And it's only in the last few decades that the mental health field (and its diagnostic classification system) has acknowledged that children don't experience psychiatric problems in the exact same way as adults—that there are developmental differences in how psychopathology manifests itself in different age groups. Numerous studies now have shown that not only do virtually all psychiatric disorders appear differently in kids and adults to some extent, but there also are differences between younger and older kids. For instance, anxious kids—

particularly younger ones—are likely to have nightmares related to their anxiety, to cling or hide, and to have stomachaches (headaches and back pain, rather than stomachaches, are more likely in anxious adults).

Some have argued that the DSM-IV changes may have been a step backwards, at least with regard to overanxious children. The move away from a separate childhood category for these young-sters, and the use of criteria derived from anxious adult patients, is reminiscent of a time years ago when psychiatry viewed children as "miniature adults." Although the DSM-IV criteria for generalized anxiety disorder do contain a "developmental modifier" for use with children—requiring only one of the six anxiety symptoms, rather than three of six, as is the case for adults—the validity of this re-mains to be determined.

Another related issue was whether kids who previously would have received a diagnosis of overanxious disorder would now meet the criteria for generalized anxiety disorder since the symptoms of the two disorders aren't exactly the same. Would some of these kids end up undiagnosed despite having significant problems with anxiety?

Let's look at the symptoms of generalized anxiety disorder to ex-plore this distinction further. Reading the sidebar on page 120, you'll see that—as for overanxious disorder—worry is a central component of GAD. Here the worry is described as anticipation that something is going to go wrong.

Although children with generalized anxiety disorder can worry about virtually anything, like Lynn, introduced at the beginning of this chapter, there is a tendency for them to worry excessively about their competence or the quality of their performance in the things they do. It should be pointed out, though, that when kids with this disorder worry about their performance, it's not about how they will appear to other people (as is the case for kids who have social anxiety disorder—see Chapter 7), it's about *how they appear to themselves*. That's why children with generalized anxiety disorder often are described as "perfectionists."

> "Perfectionist" is a label often used to describe kids with generalized anxiety disorder.

In addition to worry, children have to have at least one of six other symptoms to be diagnosed with generalized anxiety disorder. Four of the symptoms have to do with the physical effects of anxiety—feeling restless or antsy, tiring easily, having tight muscles, and having trouble with sleep (either falling asleep, staying asleep, or sleeping peacefully). Another of the symptoms focuses on the interference of anxiety with thinking and concentration, and the final one—irritability—is a mood problem that can go along with anxiety.

To receive this diagnosis, a child has to have all of the symptoms more than 50 percent of the time for a period of at least six months. And, as was the case for overanxious disorder, the symptoms can't be related exclusively to another anxiety disorder, like social phobia or separation anxiety disorder.

Are the criteria for generalized anxiety disorder better at identifying kids who are chronically, overly anxious? Even though it's been more than a decade since the switch was made from overanxious to generalized anxiety disorder, we still don't have the answer to this.

My personal impression is that generalized anxiety disorder falls short by excluding some of the frequent elements of these kids' conditions—like complaints of stomachaches and headaches and an excessive need for reassurance—that were included in overanxious disorder. Also, some of the symptoms of generalized anxiety disorder don't apply well to young children. For instance, it's relatively rare for anxious elementary-school-age kids to complain of having tense muscles or of being easily fatigued.

But putting this aside, what we do know for sure is that there are some kids—possibly including your child—who will be overlooked if only the symptoms of generalized anxiety disorder are used to arrive at a diagnosis. Research done in the late 1990s at our Florida-based child anxiety clinic at Nova Southeastern University in Fort Lauderdale showed there are children who meet the criteria for overanxious disorder but not generalized anxiety disorder. Other scientists have communicated to me that they've had similar findings, which is not surprising given that the criteria for the two disorders aren't identical.

What does all this mean for you? Well, first, if in reading this you find your son or daughter has the characteristics of *either* overanxious disorder or generalized anxiety disorder, you can be confident

Symptoms of Generalized Anxiety Disorder

The child must have the following symptom for at least half the time for six months or longer to receive this diagnosis:

- Feels overly anxious and worried (anticipating that something will go wrong) about a number of events or activities.

And at least one of the following:

- Feels restless, antsy, or wired.
- Tires easily.
- Can't concentrate or experiences mental lapses.
- Feels irritable.
- Has tight muscles.
- Has trouble falling asleep, staying asleep, or sleeping peacefully.

you're in the right chapter, the one that addresses the anxiety problems of your child. Second, you should know that some clinicians today still use the term *overanxious disorder* even though it no longer exists as an actual diagnosis. So if your doctor refers to your child's condition this way, you'll understand what he or she is talking about. Finally, if you know your child is a worrier, but the doctor says it's not an anxiety disorder, you might want to raise the issue of overanxious disorder. You certainly don't want your child's problem ignored because of an ongoing debate about how best to diagnose children like yours.

I'd like to make one last point before moving on from this topic. Although I've mentioned some difficulties you might experience because of changes in the way this anxiety disorder is diagnosed, I want to emphasize that excessive *worrying about the future* has been and continues to be key *regardless* of which diagnosis you're talking about. In fact, although this specific type of worrying is not required for the diagnosis (because kids need to have only four of the seven symptoms listed, and none of these has to be excessive worry about the future), a study we conducted in Pittsburgh (reported in the *Journal of Abnormal Child Psychology* in 1988) of fifty-five children with overanxious disorder showed that 95 percent of kids ages five to eleven had this symptom, and (as a point of interest) virtually all of the older kids did too.

> **Excessive worrying about the future is key to both overanxious and generalized anxiety disorders.**

The Many Faces of Generalized Anxiety Disorder

Although all kids with generalized anxiety disorder are, by definition, worriers, what they worry about, how they deal with their worries, and the other anxiety symptoms they have as a result of their worries aren't the same. And if we add to the mix kids who have symptoms of overanxious disorder, the variety of different ways these children can appear grows even larger.

Todd

Todd has a serious confidence problem. No matter what he's doing, he's always concerned it won't be good enough. His fourth-grade teacher says his worries don't make sense. Todd is an excellent student, the "star" of the after- school basketball team, and has outstanding musical ability—he's even been asked to play solos in the school band.

But despite his accomplishments Todd continues to worry, and it looks like his anxiety may be making him sick. He has bad headaches the doctors can't find a cause for even after many tests. He also doesn't sleep well. He tosses and turns so much through the night that he wakes up tangled in his covers or they wind up on the bedroom floor.

Todd's parents complain that he acts like he has "a chip on his shoulder"—very irritable and easily annoyed. They wish he could be more easygoing, more like their other children.

It's clear that Todd has generalized anxiety disorder. He worries excessively and needlessly (as pointed out by his teacher) about his competence in a variety of activities at school. He also is a restless sleeper and is frequently irritable, two symptoms that are very characteristic of kids with this disorder.

It looks like Todd's headaches also are related to his anxiety. Like the somatic complaints of other children with generalized anxiety disorder, Todd's headaches have no obvious pattern or relationship to any particular situation or event. That's because they're probably triggered by his worries, which he may not be entirely aware of or not sharing with his parents.

> Somatic symptoms—like headaches and stomachaches—may seem to "come out of the blue," but they're really triggered by worrying.

Todd's irritability isn't a problem at school, but his parents and siblings find he's very difficult to get along with. Hopefully, when Todd gets the help he needs, his family life will become more harmonious.

Lisa

Ten-year-old Lisa worries a lot about her health and safety. When there was a tropical storm in the Caribbean, she was sure it would become a hurricane and hit her home. After pricking her finger with a thumbtack, she worried for days that she would get "blood poisoning." She's even nervous riding in her parents' car. When her dad drives on a busy highway, she clutches her seat, certain they'll be in an accident.

Lisa is also anxious about things kids her age usually don't think about. For instance, she's already concerned about getting into a good college, even though she hasn't entered middle school yet.

In addition to, or because of, her worries, Lisa feels on edge most of the time—she's really never able to relax. She startles easily—a loud, unexpected noise sends her "through the roof." She has nervous habits too, like biting her nails and playing with her hair, twirling it around her fingers over and over again. She also has trouble with her concentration. In school she finds herself "blanking out" for no apparent reason.

Lisa's mom says her daughter has been like this ever since she can remember. She wonders, "Is this Lisa's nature, or can she really change?"

Lisa is a good example of a child who has generalized anxiety disorder. She has a lot of anxiety and worry, so much so that she's tense and on edge most of the time and has difficulty concentrating in school. Like many kids with this disorder, Lisa also has a dramatic startle response and nervous habits.

Some of Lisa's worries focus on subjects that are not appropriate for a child her age. This isn't unusual in kids with generalized anxiety disorder. The problem is that it can make them appear "hyper-mature" and interfere with their fitting in and being accepted by children their own age. Lisa, unfortunately, has experienced this. She's ostracized by the other kids in her class and has difficulty making friends.

Her mother's concern that Lisa's anxiety problem may just be "her nature" and possibly not able to be changed is a perception that's not uncommon among parents of children with generalized anxiety disorder. This is an important issue we'll address a little later on.

Sammy

Sammy's continuous worrying is driving his parents nuts. Every time he gets anxious about something, which is quite often, he turns to his mom or dad for reassurance. "Are you sure it's going to be okay?" he asks repeatedly until his folks refuse to answer him anymore. Sometimes he'll even wake them up at night when he can't fall asleep because of something he's concerned about.

Sammy's second-grade teacher also has to endure his anxious questioning. On homework, tests, even when she's just explaining something, Sammy always is the one with his hand up. She also has noticed that he's very restless, constantly fidgeting in his seat—crossing and uncrossing his legs, shifting his position in the chair, swinging his leg or tapping his foot on the ground. But in general

Sammy is very well behaved. In fact he's actually afraid of getting in trouble or doing something wrong.

Sammy definitely worries that something will go wrong, the hallmark of generalized anxiety disorder. He's almost constantly worrying about things before they happen both at home and at school. He also is restless during the day and has difficulty falling asleep at night, which are other defining features of this anxiety disorder.

Even though excessively seeking reassurance is not included in the diagnostic criteria for generalized anxiety disorder (you'll remember that it was part of overanxious disorder), it's often seen in kids with this diagnosis. Sammy definitely has this problem. His anxiety leads him to repeatedly seek reassurance from the important adults in his life. And, as is the case for many people who are close to kids like this, his parents and teacher frequently are exasperated by this behavior.

As is true for many kids with generalized anxiety disorder, Sammy's restlessness makes him look somewhat "hyper." In fact his mom wonders whether he might be hyperactive. His teacher, though, who has seen lots of kids with attention-deficit/hyperactivity disorder, doesn't think so. That's because, as we discussed in Chapter 2, the hyperactivity (and impulsivity) of kids with ADHD causes them to be disruptive and get in trouble at school. Sammy isn't like this. He's actually the opposite—very concerned about getting in trouble or doing something wrong.

Elena

Elena's kindergarten teacher is concerned. Elena needs everything to be perfect or she gets very upset. If she accidentally colors outside the lines or makes a mistake with one of her letters (for instance, writing a "d" when she means to draw a "b"), she rips up the paper and starts over again. In gym class she kicks the soccer ball against the wall if she misses a goal. She becomes tearful when she gets an answer to one of the teacher's questions wrong.

Elena also worries about things. When her mom takes her someplace she hasn't been before, she's afraid they'll get lost. After her hamster died she was worried for weeks that something was going to happen to her fish. When she was out of school for a few days for a special family vacation she was very anxious about how the teacher would react when she returned.

Elena often has stomachaches and sometimes, when she's really nervous, she throws up. Recently she has developed a really big fear of vomiting and is afraid to go places where she thinks it might happen—places where she's felt sick before.

It's obvious that Elena is overly concerned with how well she does at things. She becomes very irritated when she thinks she has made a mistake or failed in some way. Because of this, her mom and teacher describe her as a "perfectionist," a label that, as I mentioned earlier, is often applied to kids like this. Elena's also a worrier and fearful when it comes to many things, like her physical well-being (getting in an accident; throwing up), potential losses (her pets), and how authority figures (her teacher) perceive her.

As I mention in the sidebar on the next page, it's not unusual for kids like Elena—kids who have generalized anxiety disorder—to develop phobias. In fact it looks like Elena's fear of vomiting is heading in this direction.

Elena is a good example of a young child who is overly anxious, but she doesn't meet the criteria for generalized anxiety disorder quite as clearly as the other children I've just described. She probably would have fit the older overanxious disorder criteria better, and because of this change it's possible she might be overlooked and go undiagnosed if she was evaluated for an anxiety disorder at this time. That certainly would be a shame since this really is the best time to turn things around for her.

Is This Really an Anxiety Disorder?

Because generalized anxiety disorder usually starts young and tends to persist, and the symptoms of the disorder are so pervasive, affecting many aspects of children's lives, it's sometimes mistaken for an anxious "personality style" rather than an anxiety disorder. Like Lisa's mom, you or your spouse may interpret your child's symptoms like this, or you may run into professionals who do.

Facts about Generalized Anxiety Disorder

Although generalized anxiety disorder usually *starts early*, kids rarely receive professional help for it before they're adolescents.

The families of children with generalized anxiety disorder tend to be at *higher income levels*.

The disorder tends to be *chronic*, but isn't always the same. It's typical for kids to have periods when they're relatively better and other times when they're worse.

Most children with generalized anxiety have, or will develop, *another anxiety disorder* too.

The most common additional anxiety disorder is a specific or social *phobia*.

Depression is not uncommon in kids with generalized anxiety, especially once they've reached puberty.

A personality style—of any type—does not produce the levels of distress that psychiatric disorders do, or interfere with day-to-day functioning. Just look at the kids I talked about in the last few pages. All four of them are experiencing a lot of discomfort, and their symptoms have caused problems with their school, home, or social lives.

Viewing the symptoms of generalized anxiety disorder as personality traits rather than part of an anxiety disorder can keep your child from getting the help he or she needs. Not only does this mean your child continues to suffer now; it also can have major consequences for your child's future. That's because the disorder does not, in most cases, go away on its own. To the contrary, it usually gets worse as kids get older, and they often develop other anxiety disorders or depression. That's why it's so important that you and your child *get a handle on this now*.

If you are concerned that your child may have generalized anxiety disorder and your doctor minimizes or dismisses the problem, you might want to consider getting a second opinion, particularly from someone who specializes in childhood anxiety disorders.

"I Don't Want to Go!": Generalized Anxiety and Avoidance Behavior

In Chapters 1 and 2 we talked about how avoidance behavior is a defining feature of many of the childhood anxiety disorders. You may have noticed, though, from the sidebar on page 120, that it's not included as one of the symptoms of generalized anxiety disorder. The symptoms of generalized anxiety disorder focus more on thoughts (worries) and feelings (the physiological aspects of anxiety) than on behavior.

However, if your child has generalized anxiety disorder, there undoubtedly will be times when he or she tries to get out of doing something or going somewhere because of anxiety. That's avoidance behavior, and for many kids it shows up in relation to school.

Children with generalized anxiety disorder usually don't have really severe problems with school absenteeism (unlike children with separation anxiety disorder, who can miss months or even years of school), but your child may resist going when faced with a stressful event or situation or on occasions where there is a concern about "performance" in some way. Let me give you a few examples of this so you can see what I mean.

Kids may resist going to school when they're worried about some aspect of their school performance.

Eleven-year-old Josh is a perfectionist. He always puts a lot of time into his homework to make sure it's just right. But last night his Little League game ran longer than expected and he wasn't able to give his assignment the attention it needed. The next morning when it was time to get up for school he told his mom, "I don't want to go."

Thatcher, a fourth grader with generalized anxiety disorder, gets extremely anxious about tests. If he's feeling really insecure about how he's going to do—because he doesn't think he's prepared enough or the subject matter is really tough—he pleads to stay home.

Five-year-old Sadie is worried she didn't pick the right thing for show-and-tell. When her mom wakes her up to go to school, Sadie tells her, "I have a tummy ache" and won't get out of bed.

Although kids like Josh, Thatcher, and Sadie try to avoid school at times, in general they, like other children with generalized anxiety disorder, don't want to miss school. Absences from school usually *increase* anxiety for kids with this disorder because it's so important to them to stay on top of their work. They also don't want to fall out of favor with their teachers by having unexplained or questionable absences. (You'll remember Sammy and Elena—described earlier in this chapter—who also were afraid of their teachers' disapproval. Like them, kids with generalized anxiety disorder frequently are overconcerned about how they're perceived by authority figures— other than their parents—and super well behaved around them.)

Your child may try to avoid other situations besides school. Ten-year-old Louis, who is somewhat uncoordinated, shies away from participating in sports because he's concerned he won't do well. Candace, a first grader, wants to drop out of ballet class because she's worried about the upcoming recital.

Louis and Candace want to avoid situations where they're concerned about their performance. The children who tried to get out of going to school had performance-related anxiety too. But avoidance behavior isn't always fueled by fears about performance.

Yolanda's mom says her daughter is extremely anxious in new situations, much more so than other kids her age. She resists going places she hasn't been before, even to do fun things like Brownies and day camp.

Yolanda is like a lot of other kids with generalized anxiety disorder. They're uncomfortable in—and often try to avoid—new situations because the unfamiliarity increases their apprehensive expectation. This is one of the problems we'll talk about in the next section, where we get into how to tackle the different aspects of generalized anxiety disorder.

Overcoming Generalized Anxiety Disorder

As I said at the very beginning of this chapter, generalized anxiety disorder definitely is an anxiety disorder that should be nipped in the bud. Because it tends to be chronic—going from childhood to adolescence and then adolescence into adulthood, and usually gets worse as your child gets older—your best chance of helping your child is to address the problem *now*.

In this section I've given you the steps you need to help your child overcome generalized anxiety disorder. While many parents will be able to use this information successfully by itself, without the assistance of a mental health professional, there are some circumstances where this may not be the best way to proceed.

Eight-year-old Sawyer's sleep is so bad he can hardly function at school. He can't concentrate in class, and the teacher says he often falls asleep with his head on his desk. Emma, a fourth grader, is so anxious and agitated that she feels like she's jumping out of her skin. She can't sit still and feels compelled to pace. Connie, age ten, is tormented by nonstop worries. She goes to her folks for reassurance thirty to forty times a day.

If your son or daughter has severe symptoms of generalized anxiety disorder—like Sawyer, Emma, or Connie—you probably shouldn't tackle things completely on your own. Consider taking your child to a doctor who specializes in childhood anxiety disorders, at least for an evaluation. That way you'll know if professional treatment is indicated. If this is the case, you still can work with your child at home using the strategies here, but be sure first to share the information in this section with the doctor to make sure both of you are "on the same page."

1. Pay attention to your child's diet, activity level, and sleep habits.

Consider the role of diet.

In Chapter 3 I talked about several aspects of your child's diet that can play a role in creating anxiety. While attending to these things is important for kids with any type of anxiety disorder, it's especially critical for children who have generalized anxiety disorder. Because kids with this disorder usually have persistently high levels of physiological arousal, you don't want them to ingest anything that can increase these levels even more.

Foods and beverages that contain caffeine or sugar can do this. Caffeine is a stimulant drug that produces anxiety symptoms. It also can trigger hypoglycemic reactions by first increasing your child's blood sugar level and then sending it plummeting. Sugar can create hypoglycemic reactions in the same way. Hypoglycemic reactions, as you'll recall from Chapter 3, frequently have anxiety symptoms as a component.

Try to keep caffeine and sugar out of your child's diet as best you can. Take another look at Chapter 3 (including the chart on the caffeine content of common foods and beverages your child is likely to be consuming) for suggestions on how to do this. In addition, try to make sure your child doesn't skip meals and that he or she eats between-meal snacks. This also will reduce the likelihood of low blood sugar levels and hypoglycemic reactions.

It's also a good idea to be on the lookout for food allergies or sensitivities, which can worsen your child's anxiety. If you suspect your child has food allergies, find out what they are (visit a pediatric allergist who can test for them) and remove the allergens from your child's diet.

Is Your Child's Diet Part of the Problem?

	Yes	No
Does your child consume a lot of high-*caffeine* foods or beverages, like chocolate, certain sodas, or iced tea?	☐	☐
Does your child's diet include a lot of *sugar*? Does he or she regularly eat candy, cake, cookies, or ice cream?	☐	☐
Does he or she *skip meals*? Almost never eat snacks?	☐	☐
Do you suspect that your child may have *food allergies*?	☐	☐
Do you think your child may be sensitive to *chemicals* contained in foods, like preservatives, dyes, or other artificial ingredients?	☐	☐

Checking "yes" to any of these questions means that diet may be contributing to your child's anxiety problem.

Unfortunately, there are no tests for sensitivities to the chemicals that are contained in many of our foods and beverages, so if you think your child has this problem (which, as we discussed in Chapter 3, can cause anxiety symptoms), the best thing to do is to eliminate dyes, preservatives, and other artificial ingredients for a couple of weeks and observe the results. Luckily today this is not nearly as difficult as it once was. Most supermarkets have organic sections, and there are specialty grocery stores (some of which are chains) entirely devoted to these types of foods.

Ensure that your child is physically active.

There's absolutely no question about the value of physical activity in reducing anxiety. And since kids with generalized anxiety disorder are anxious much (if not all) of the time, it's especially important for them. In fact if your child has this anxiety disorder, *daily* exercise is what you should be aiming for.

Activities that are aerobic—that increase heart rate for a sustained period of time (optimally, twenty minutes)—are particularly good for your child because they decrease "baseline," or "resting," levels of anxiety. I've included a few examples of aerobic activities in the sidebar on the next page, but there are many others besides these.

Don't be limited by the idea that physical activity has to fall under the category of "exercise" to be effective. As you can see, I've listed several sports and recreational activities that wouldn't be considered "exercise" according to the common usage of this word. There also are household chores kids can take part in—like helping their moms or dads rake leaves or vacuum—that can have aerobic benefits.

Physical activity can have other positive effects on your child's mental health besides reducing anxiety. Gil, a third grader with generalized anxiety and a self-esteem problem, started taking karate in the fall. As he practiced and became more proficient at his karate skills, his self-confidence improved as well.

Gymnastics, martial arts, ballet, and other physical activities that emphasize controlled movement are particularly helpful in building kids' self-confidence. If your child has a confidence problem, as

Aerobic Activities

Basketball	Jogging	Skateboarding
Bicycling	Jumping rope	Skiing
Dancing	Roller blading	Soccer
Ice skating	Running	Swimming

many kids with generalized anxiety disorder do, consider getting him or her involved in one of these activities. You may be surprised by how much your child gains.

Make certain your child gets enough sleep.

As we saw earlier, sleep problems are common in kids who have generalized anxiety disorder. The trouble with reduced sleep or poor-quality sleep, in addition to its effects on physical health, is that it can end up increasing your child's anxiety. When children do not get enough rest, their "defenses are down" and they're more prone to apprehensive expectation.

Good "sleep hygiene" (see the sidebar on the facing page) will go a long way toward helping your child get a good night's sleep. Pay attention to what your child eats and drinks in the evening, activities engaged in before bedtime, and your child's sleep environment, and you'll see what a big difference this makes. Also setting (and enforcing!) a regular bedtime is very important. You aren't doing your child a favor by allowing him or her to stay up late to watch television or use the computer.

Sydney, a sixth grader with generalized anxiety disorder, is at the age where she's self-conscious about being overweight. She's started doing sit-ups and push-ups right before bedtime, trying to burn calories and lose weight. But Sydney's finding she's having a hard time falling asleep—sometimes it takes her more than an hour before she drifts off.

Although I strongly encourage exercise and physical activity for kids with generalized anxiety disorder, Sydney has picked the very worst time to do this. Getting her "adrenaline pumping" at bedtime is interfering with her ability to fall asleep, which, in turn, probably will make her anxiety worse the next day (and could also lead to more overeating, since kids—and adults too for that matter—may overeat in response to anxiety and stress.)

If your child has a severe sleep problem, the suggestions I've given may not be enough. In that case you may want to talk to your child's pediatrician about nutritional supplements or over-the-counter and prescription medications that are available, or consider going to a mental health professional for help.

2. Help your child develop better ways of looking at things.

Most kids with generalized anxiety disorder anticipate "the worst" even when there's no evidence to support their fears. To eliminate their worries and anxiety they need to look at alternative possible outcomes that are more reasonable and optimistic. One way parents

Getting a Good Night's Sleep

Set and enforce a *regular bedtime* **and** a regular wake-up time. If your child has difficulty falling or staying asleep, don't allow naps during the day.

Don't let your child engage in anything mentally, emotionally, or physically taxing (homework; a scary movie; exercise) within an hour of bedtime. Instead, *wind down* with relaxing—not stimulating—activities.

Bed should be for sleep only, not for other activities.

Avoid *foods or beverages that contain caffeine or sugar* after 4:00 P.M.

An *evening snack* that has protein and carbohydrate—like cheese and crackers or peanut butter on toast—can help your child *stay* asleep. Foods that contain the amino acid tryptophan (found in milk and turkey) are good for *inducing* sleep.

Limiting your child's *fluid intake* after 7:00 P.M. will cut down on trips to the bathroom during the night.

Make sure your child is *comfortable* with the right sleepwear and bedcovers (cotton is best), mattress, and room temperature. If your child has allergies, ask your doctor what you can do to make your child's bedroom more allergy-proof.

can help with this is by demonstrating healthy thinking for their children.

Nine-year-old Kylie is worried about going to her friend's birthday party tomorrow. Even though she's a very likable kid who gets along well with other children, she's concerned that she doesn't know most of the kids who will be there. When she tells her mom, "I won't have anyone to talk to or play with," her mom replies, "This will be a good opportunity to make new friends. Whenever you meet new kids your age you usually get along with them great!"

Mariah, a fifth grader, is worried she's not going to do a good enough job on her school paper. Her mom says, "You always get excellent grades on your papers—there's no reason this time will be any different!"

Both of these moms have shown their daughters alternative, and more realistic, ways of thinking about situations they're worried about, ways that are less likely to make them anxious. When your child anticipates a negative outcome to an upcoming event, like Kylie's and Mariah's moms, you too should step in and offer a more reasonable and positive point of view.

Another more structured way to help your child with negative anticipation is to use the list approach. The technique involves having your child identify the negative outcome he or she anticipates and then come up with at least three possible more reasonable, alternative outcomes.

To get an idea how this is done, let's use the example of a birthday party again, but this time it's eleven-year-old Keiko's party and she's afraid the kids she invited won't show up. Using the form on the facing page, Keiko writes on the top of the page "No one is going to show up at my party." Then, under that, she lists other possible outcomes—more rational alternatives:

1. Most of the kids probably will show up because their mothers called and said they were coming.
2. Even if some of the kids don't come to the party, the rest of us still can have a good time.
3. All of these kids came to my birthday party last year and had a great time. There's no reason it should be different this year.

My Worries: Better Ways to Look at Things

What I'm worried will happen:

_____

_____

_____

_____

Other ways to think about it:

1. _____

_____

_____

_____

2. _____

_____

_____

_____

3. _____

_____

_____

_____

Keiko was able to come up with three more optimistic—and probable—outcomes. Once she did this, she no longer was worried about her party.

Remember Lisa, the girl who was afraid a tropical storm was going to become a hurricane and hit her home? She used the list technique and this is what she came up with:

1. The tropical storm may not become a hurricane.
2. The storm may become a hurricane that doesn't cause big damage.
3. The storm may become a hurricane but head away from my home.

Like Keiko, Lisa was able to decrease her negative anticipation (that in this case really was quite catastrophic) by thinking of and focusing on several less devastating potential outcomes. In fact the technique was so successful that she was able to completely forget about the storm.

Your child can fill out the form for any worry that becomes problematic; extra copies of the form are at the back of the book.

If you are a very anxious person, or even have generalized anxiety disorder yourself, you may have a hard time helping your child with the methods I've just discussed. In this case you probably will need to work on how you look at things first before you can assist your child. There are many books available that can show you how to go about doing this, and you also can use the list technique included here. Or you may decide to see a cognitive therapist who specializes in teaching people how to modify their thoughts.

If you don't want to tackle your own problems at this time but you do want your child to get help with negative anticipation, there's always the option of having your son or daughter see a professional to work on this. What's important is that your child learns to look at things in a healthier manner, not how he or she gets that way.

3. Help your child get control over worrying by using the scheduling approach.

One of the most difficult aspects of excessive worrying for your child is the feeling of having little or no control over it. Worrying by definition is intrusive and persistent and can't easily be put aside. But literally scheduling worrying—that is, having a specific period of time set aside during the day for worrying—helps many children gain that sense of control. The technique can be used alone or in combination with the list approach we just discussed.

To use this technique, you and your child first will need to select a short period of time that will be set aside each day as the time to worry. I recommend anywhere from five to thirty minutes, depending on the age of your child but on other factors too (like how many worries are present, the severity of the worries, the ability of the child to sustain attention on a task, maturity, and intellectual level). As a general rule, children who are five or six will do well with a five- or ten- minute time period, seven or eight with ten to fifteen minutes, nine or ten with fifteen to twenty minutes, and eleven or twelve with twenty to thirty minutes.

The best time usually is during the early evening after dinner and once homework has been completed, but not before bedtime when it could affect your child's sleep.

Once you've settled on a time period, pick a quiet place where the worrying will be done. There are many places that can work well for this; just make sure your child doesn't use his or her bed (you don't want there to be an association between worrying and being in bed, or your child could develop trouble falling asleep). For the technique to be most effective, your child should use the same spot and same time period every day.

Keisha, age eight, schedules her worrying. At 7:00 each night she sits at the kitchen table and talks with her mom about what's worrying her. Ten-year-old Preston likes to use the list method. Before he watches his evening TV shows he's at his desk coming up with other ways to look at things that have been troubling him.

You can be with your child during the worry period, like Keisha's mom, to provide information, offer support, and be a general "sounding board." But if you do this, please make sure you don't inadvertently respond to requests for reassurance (see strategy 5, below). Don't answer any question more than once, and remember that you can encourage your child to use the list approach (see strategy 2, above) with the form on page 135 to come up with thoughts to combat the worries.

When upsetting thoughts occur outside of the worry period, your child should try to cut off the worry as soon as possible by saying (silently if with other people, out loud if alone) "I'll worry about that later—during my worry time." Sometimes children have to say this two or three times before they're successful at putting a worry aside. But as they become more used to doing this once usually is enough.

There are many benefits to scheduling worry. As I said earlier, it helps children feel they have control over the problem. Also, confining worrying to a specific period of time cuts down on the distress your child is likely to experience during the day and lessens its effects on your child's daily activities.

> **Scheduling worrying helps kids feel they have control over their worries rather than their worrying controlling them.**

There's one more potential benefit from using this technique that I'd like to mention before we move on to our next topic. Some kids are successful at pushing away their worries during the day but find that when they try to produce them during the worry period *they're not able to* (there is actually a type of psychotherapy—called "paradoxical intention"—based on the premise that people can't bring on their own symptoms at will or "on demand"). So if you find your child is having this experience using the scheduling approach, you'll know the reason for what you're seeing and that you should just be glad of it—these kids effectively eliminate worrying throughout their days, just like the kids who are able to summon up worries during a scheduled time period.

4. Teach your child relaxation skills to decrease the physical aspects of anxiety.

Although they show it in different ways (feeling on edge; physical restlessness; nervous habits), all children with generalized anxiety disorder have elevated levels of physiological arousal. Earlier, when we talked about diet and exercise, I pointed out how important it is to bring this level down.

Deep muscle relaxation, a relaxation method widely used for treating anxiety disorders, does this. It not only alleviates muscle tension, as its name implies, it also decreases other physical aspects of anxiety and lowers your child's overall arousal level.

The technique involves tightening and then relaxing different muscles in the body. Nine exercises are done in sequence, each one targeting a different muscle group. Each exercise is done twice before moving on to the next. In total they take about ten to fifteen minutes to complete.

It's a good idea for you to familiarize yourself with the exercises first and then teach them to your child. Your child needs to be lying down in a quiet place to do them. Bed is fine for this, but be aware that some kids fall asleep while doing the exercises. This is good if your child has difficulty falling asleep, as long as it's done at bedtime (as I mentioned in the sidebar on page 133, naps during the day can worsen sleep problems). If your child wears glasses or contacts, please make sure they're removed. Also, kids should be wearing comfortable, nonrestrictive clothing when they do the exercises.

1. Clench your *left fist* very tightly. Hold and concentrate on the tension in your fist and your arm (*for about 10 seconds*). Now relax the fist and the arm, resting your arm in your lap or on the bed (*relax for about 20 seconds*). Now, once again, clench your left fist very tightly (*hold the tension for about 10 seconds*). Relax, letting your arm drop to your side (*remain relaxed for about 20 seconds*).
2. Now do the same with the *right fist*. Clench the right fist really tight and notice the tension in your fist and your arm (*hold for about 10 seconds*). Relax the fist and the arm, letting it rest comfortably in your lap or on the bed (*relax for about 20 seconds*). Now repeat the exercise.
3. Now, *bend both hands back at the wrists* with your fingers pointing toward the ceiling. Feel the tense muscles in the back of your hand and in your lower arms (*hold for about 10 seconds*). Now relax your hands and let them fall to your sides (*relax for about 20 seconds*). Repeat.
4. Now, clench both of your hands into *fists and bring them toward your shoulders*, so that the upper parts of your arms are tense. Hold the tension (*for about 10 seconds*). Now let go of the tension and relax, letting your arms fall to your sides (*relax for about 20 seconds*). Repeat.

5. Next, *shrug your shoulders*, bringing both shoulders up toward your ears, as if you were going to touch your ears with your shoulders. Hold your shoulders like that (*for about 10 seconds*) and feel the tension in your neck and in your shoulders. Now relax, letting your arms drop onto the bed (*relax for about 20 seconds*). Repeat.

6. Now *close your eyes very tightly*, so tightly that you can feel the tension all around your eyes. Hold the tension (*for about 10 seconds*). Now let go and relax the muscles (*relax for about 20 seconds*). Repeat.

7. Now take a really *deep breath*, filling your lungs, and hold it (*for about 10 seconds*). Exhale and continue breathing as you were (*relax like this for about 20 seconds*). Repeat.

8. Next, *stretch both legs straight out,* pointing your toes. Stretch them as much as you can so that you feel tension in your upper legs (*hold for about 10 seconds*). Now relax your legs, letting all the tension go (*relax for about 20 seconds*). Repeat.

9. Now *tense both legs by pointing your toes upward*, toward your head. Feel the tension in the muscles of your lower legs (*hold for about 10 seconds*). Now relax, letting all the tension go (*remain relaxed for about 20 seconds*). Repeat.

Children should practice the exercises at least once a day for a couple of weeks to get really familiar with them. Then they can be used as needed. Since the exercises don't take very long to do, kids often do them whenever they're feeling especially tense or nervous (there's no limit on the number of times they can be done in a day). As I said earlier, they also can be used as a sleep aid at bedtime.

Nine-year-old Collin likes to do the exercises when he comes home from school and is feeling wound up from the day's events. Mercedes, age eleven, always feels uptight the night before tests. She finds using the relaxation technique helps get rid of her anxiety.

Even though Collin and Mercedes use the relaxation exercises selectively as they need them, I believe that, like physical exercise, it's very helpful for kids with generalized anxiety disorder to do them on a daily basis, regardless of how they're feeling. If you can incorporate this into your child's daily schedule (like every evening at bedtime or each day after school), I know you'll see the rewards.

5. Decrease requests for reassurance and increase your child's self-confidence.

Like Sammy, introduced earlier, many kids with generalized anxiety disorder repeatedly seek reassurance from the important adults in their life, such as their parents and teachers, about situations they're anxious and worried about. Children's concerns about their safety ("Will I be okay?"), their competence ("Will I do okay?"), their capacity to make decisions and avoid making mistakes ("Is this the right thing to do?"), and their ability to handle different situations ("Will I be able to do this?"), lead them to ask the same questions over and over again even though the answers they get don't change.

When your child gets reassurance from you, his or her anxiety immediately is reduced. Unfortunately, though, the anxiety reduction "reinforces" or strengthens the tendency to seek reassurance, and that's why your child continues to ask the same question again and again. (As you'll see in Chapter 6, this is similar to the way obsessions and compulsions become repetitive.)

To develop self-confidence, and overcome generalized anxiety disorder, children must learn to get control of their worries and *reassure themselves* using one of the methods discussed earlier. But before they can do this parents need a new way to handle their children's excessive requests for reassurance.

Generally speaking the best way to respond to requests for reassurance is *not* to respond to them, that is, to ignore them. I know this sounds rough, but keep in mind that you aren't helping your child by continuously answering the same questions. Please also keep in mind that what I'm talking about here is repetitive, often relentless, reassurance seeking ("Mommy, are you sure it's going to be all right?" . . . "Are you absolutely sure it's going to be all right?" . . . "Mom, are you sure?" . . . "Are you sure?" and so on), not legitimate concerns that children genuinely need to have addressed.

How do you know whether your child's question is going to be a single legitimate request for information or support or whether it's just the first of

> **The best way to respond to excessive requests for reassurance is _not_ to respond to them.**

many to follow? Unless you know the areas your child tends to be insecure and repetitive about, or you've addressed the same issue in the past, it's probably not going to be possible to know this in advance. That's why I suggest that you *answer your child's initial question but ignore any subsequent questions that ask the same thing* (even if they're worded somewhat differently, but really are attempts to get a response to the same issue). If you're not comfortable with completely ignoring the additional questions you can respond once—and only once—with "I already answered that." Please *do not* make the mistake of saying this every time your child asks you the same question, or you'll end up getting *even more* questions (in this case your attention, not anxiety reduction, is reinforcing the behavior).

Tell your child, in a very clear but emphatic manner, how you are going to be handling the repetitive questioning from now on *before* you begin using this new procedure. It's also a good idea to start tackling requests for reassurance after children have learned the techniques for managing worry so they already have in place other (better) ways to deal with them. Finally, it's smart to include your child's teacher in what you're planning on doing. Chances are that if your son or daughter is showing this problem at home the teacher also is seeing it at school. Having consistency in how requests for reassurance are addressed will help ensure your child gets past this problem.

Reducing requests for reassurance increases children's self-confidence because kids are forced to rely on their own resources and skills for managing their worries. There's another aspect of generalized anxiety disorder, though, that also can undermine your child's self-confidence. Let's turn to this now.

6. Encourage your child to try new things.

Remember Yolanda, the girl who worried about and avoided new situations? Other kids with generalized anxiety disorder also have this problem. That's because their apprehensive expectations are heightened in unfamiliar circumstances.

Joaquin, an eight-year-old with generalized anxiety disorder, is reluctant to take part in activities he hasn't participated in before.

His mom has tried to get him to join Cub Scouts or Little League, but he refuses to go to either.

What can Joaquin's mom do to get her child to try new things? One thing she can do is to *make the unfamiliar more familiar* by exposing her son to different aspects of the situation beforehand. For example, Joaquin could just observe a scout meeting or softball game to see what goes on there. He also could talk to kids he knows who take part in these activities to find out more about them. (In fact taking on a new activity where he already has friends will make going a lot easier because this too will decrease the unfamiliarity of the situation.) Another thing Joaquin's mom could do is to help him see the new experience in positive terms—"Joaquin, this will be an adventure!"—or in a way that will minimize her child's perception of risk: "Joaquin, try it once, and then if you don't like it you don't have to do it again" (for kids a couple years older than Joaquin, referring to this as "an experiment" often is very effective).

It's important to reward your child's attempts at trying new things. I talked about the use of tangible rewards in Chapter 4 (see pages 112–113), but praise alone often works equally well for kids with generalized anxiety disorder because of their "need to please." Praise your child often and as soon as possible for participating in a new activity or going someplace that's unfamiliar.

When Joaquin finally joined Little League, he saw that his worries were unfounded. This helped him develop the confidence to face other new situations in the future. Your child can become more self-confident like Joaquin. Follow the guidelines I've outlined in this section and see the positive results for yourself.

The key to conquering generalized anxiety is for children to get control of their worries. In this chapter I've included several techniques that will help your child do this, along with relaxation exercises to decrease the physical aspects of anxiety and methods for building self-confidence. Armed with these skills, you now have everything you need to help your child overcome this anxiety disorder.

6 OVER AND OVER AGAIN
Obsessive–Compulsive Disorder

Eight-year-old Brenner has an unusual habit his parents don't understand. He touches things for no apparent reason. When he walks through a doorway, he has to touch the door's frame or the knob. He also reaches out to touch any furniture he passes that's within a few feet of him.

Brenner knows his behavior looks strange, so at school and with his friends he tries to hide the touching or not do it at all. But at home it's really gotten out of control. He spends so much time at it he ends up being late for most everything.

When his parents try to stop him from touching things, Brenner gets very upset. What they don't know is that he has to do it. He's certain that if he doesn't, something really terrible will happen to his family.

Although obsessive–compulsive disorder (OCD) has been recognized in adults for more than a century, it's only fairly recently that mental health professionals have realized this psychiatric problem also occurs in children.

Researchers first began suspecting that the disorder could have a childhood onset from the histories given by adults with obsessive–compulsive disorder, who often reported that their symptoms began prior to adolescence. Following this, during the last two decades, many research studies were conducted on children with OCD, the results of which ended up drawing a lot of media attention (TV shows, magazine articles). As a result people now are much more aware of this problem, and today obsessive–compulsive disorder is often first is recognized in children by parents, teachers, pediatricians, and others who aren't in the mental health field.

It's important to differentiate the obsessions and compulsions of obsessive–compulsive disorder from normal occasional upsetting thoughts or mental images that don't make sense and from behaviors that kids (and adults too for that matter) may repeat on a limited basis. For example, normal kids may check their alarm clocks once, or even twice, before going to sleep on school nights, even though they know they've already set them.

Obsessions and compulsions are different. They are repetitive and relentless and have significant effects on kids' lives. They cause a lot of distress, frequently take up a good deal of time, and interfere with different aspects of day-to-day functioning. They can negatively impact schoolwork, friendships, out-of-school activities, and your child's overall ability to follow a normal routine (like Brenner, who is late for almost everything).

Obsessive–compulsive disorder virtually never gets better on its own. Although it may *appear* at times to be better because the nature of this disorder is to "wax and wane" (have periods when symptoms are worse and those when they're better), obsessive–compulsive disorder tends to be chronic, especially when it begins in childhood. That's why it's so critical to intervene as early as possible, so your child can learn the skills needed to bring this problem under control.

Later in this chapter we'll spend a lot of time discussing in detail the specific measures that can be used to do this. But before we get to that, let's talk about how the disorder is diagnosed to make sure your child really has this problem.

Diagnosing Obsessive–Compulsive Disorder

The symptoms of obsessive–compulsive disorder are listed in the sidebar on page 147. As you can see, to receive this diagnosis your child must have either obsessions *or* compulsions (or both).

Obsessions are intrusive, recurring thoughts or mental images that cause your child extreme anxiety or distress. But unlike worries, they are not about real-life problems and situations. The con-

tent of obsessions is inappropriate and disturbing, and kids often
are scared, repulsed, or confused
by them. To give you a better
idea of what they're like, let's
look at some children who have
this problem.

> **Unlike worries, obsessions aren't about real-life problems. They are inappropriate thoughts that don't make sense.**

- Brenner, the boy who touches things, has a very disturbing picture that keeps popping into his mind—he sees his family being burned in a fire.
- Although she has perfect eyesight, Trisha, a fifth grader, can't stop thinking that something is wrong with her eyes and that she's going to go blind.
- Nine-year-old Royce has an obsession that his hands are contaminated with germs.
- Thai, age ten, has sacrilegious thoughts that seem to come out of nowhere.
- Eleven-year-old Eduardo has inappropriate sexual images that keep entering her head.
- Although she loves her little sister, eight-year-old Meredith imagines herself harming her.

As you can see, the themes of obsessions often have to do with being harmed or doing harm, or they have unacceptable religious or sexual content. Because the content of obsessions is so distasteful, kids usually experience them as "ego-dystonic"—although they know the thoughts are theirs (and not put in their heads from some outside force), they don't view them as part of their true selves. That's why some children come up with names for their obsessive–compulsive disorder, to differentiate it—the disorder—from themselves.

Obsessions always initially cause anxiety or distress, but the level of discomfort they trigger can lessen over time. Obsessions also differ in how often they occur (their frequency) and how long they go on (their duration). Some kids have brief but frequent thoughts or mental images, while others have ones that occur less often but persist for a longer period of time. (Later on you'll see

Symptoms
of Obsessive–Compulsive Disorder

To be diagnosed with this disorder, a child must have either obsessions <u>or</u> compulsions:

Obsessions:

- Has thoughts or mental images that come back over and over that feel intrusive and inappropriate, causing extreme anxiety or distress.

- Tries to ignore or suppress the thoughts or images or "neutralize" or "undo" them with some other thought or action.

Compulsions:

- Feels the need to perform certain repeated behaviors or mental acts repeatedly in response to an obsession or according to rigid rules.

- Performs the behaviors or mental acts in an attempt to prevent or reduce distress or to prevent some dreaded event from occurring, even though the behaviors or mental acts have no realistic connection with what they're designed to "undo" or prevent or they are obviously excessive.

- Feels highly distressed by the compulsions, or the compulsions take more than one hour a day or significantly interfere with the child's normal routine, schoolwork, or social activities or relationships.

how these differences indicate which approach you and your child should take to get rid of obsessions.)

Despite these differences, all kids react to their obsessions by trying to ignore or suppress them or "neutralize" or counteract them with some other thought or action. When another thought or action is used, it usually ends up being a compulsion.

Kids often respond to obsessions with mental rituals or compulsive behaviors.

Compulsions, also referred to as *rituals*, are repetitive behaviors or mental acts kids are driven to perform in response to an obsession or according to very specific and rigid rules (see the sidebar above). Hand washing, checking, touching, tapping, redoing actions, sniffing of the hands, blinking, and grimacing are examples of behaviors that may be performed in response to obsessions.

Eight-year-old Sheldon reacts to his obsession by tapping things—his desk, the kitchen table, and any other flat surface he comes into contact with—three times (it's three because it's his "lucky number"). When Savannah, age six, has her upsetting thought, she keeps blinking until it goes away. Kirk, a third grader with an obsession about germs, turns doorknobs using the side of his hand. Avoidance rituals like Kirk's are another kind of compulsion that can be triggered by an obsession, usually a contamination-related one.

Scarlet and Bobby also have rituals they do in reaction to obsessions, but theirs are mental and can't be observed. Scarlet, age ten, has to say a prayer in her head every time she has her obsession. Bobby, a third grader, must silently count to ten when he has his "bad thought."

Some kids have compulsions without obsessions (this isn't uncommon, although the reverse—obsessions without compulsions—is). These rituals often involve arranging objects or overattention to symmetry, as for Joy, a first grader, who has to have her dolls arranged in a special way—from largest to smallest and according to hair color—and for Jerry, who makes sure all of his steps are exactly even when he walks.

Compulsions are aimed at preventing or reducing anxiety or distress (sometimes in response to an obsession) or preventing or undoing some dreaded situation (almost always a situation contained in an obsession). For example, kids who have obsessions about germs (like Kirk) or other contamination-related obsessions frequently are compulsive hand washers. The washing reduces anxiety because (in the minds of those who do it) it gets rid of or "undoes" the contamination. By contrast, children who have checking rituals usually are trying to prevent something terrible from happening rather than undoing something that already has happened.

This was the case with eleven-year-old Camille. Camille has an obsession that someone is going to break into her home and hurt her family. She repeatedly checks the locks on all the doors and windows before she goes to bed at night.

Does Your Child Have Any of These Compulsions?

Washing: Excessive washing (hand washing, bathing, or showering) or an elaborate pattern of washing that takes a long time to complete. Hand sniffing is another common compulsion seen in children that may be associated with hand washing.

Arranging objects: Having to have possessions—like stuffed animals, toy cars, books and papers on a desk—lined up symmetrically or arranged in a certain order or specific way.

Personal symmetry: Having to have things on one's body (the direction of hair on both arms), parts of the body (both feet lined up straight), or body movements (such as foot steps) symmetrical or exactly the same.

Checking: Repeatedly checking something to "make sure" an action was done, like checking that water faucets or lights are turned off, that the bedroom window is locked, that the hairdryer has been turned off or unplugged.

Redoing: Redoing the same action a certain number of times for no apparent reason, like walking in and out of a doorway several times or rereading or repeating sentences. In some cases the number of repetitions are based on "lucky" numbers.

Avoidance rituals: Avoiding coming into contact with something or someone that's thought to be contaminated in a specific (AIDS, a bodily secretion) or less specific ("cooties," germs, dirt) way. Some avoidance rituals aren't related to contamination fears (for example, avoiding walking on cracks in the sidewalk or the spaces between floor tiles).

Touching: Having to touch something once or repeatedly, usually as an (irrational) attempt to prevent something catastrophic from happening.

Vocal and ocular rituals: Attempts to suppress or neutralize an obsession by humming, grimacing, or blinking.

Mental compulsions: Acts that are performed silently, like praying, counting, or saying certain words or sentences in one's head, often as an attempt to undo or neutralize an obsessive thought.

Compulsions, by definition, either are clearly excessive—as for Camille—or not connected in a realistic way with what they're designed to undo or prevent, as when kids tap, touch, or have mental rituals in response to obsessions. It's parents, though, not children, who recognize this is the case. When asked if their compulsions don't make sense or are a problem, kids often answer "no." (This is the one way the disorder tends to differ in children and adults—adults with obsessive–compulsive disorder usually acknowledge that their behavior is extreme or unreasonable.)

Unlike obsessions, compulsions may or may not cause your child distress. However, if they don't, to be considered compulsions they must either be time-consuming (take up at least an hour a day) or have other significant effects on your child's life—like interfering with schoolwork or relationships or the ability to engage in social activities or follow a normal routine. (That's why the example of occasional checking behavior I gave at the beginning of this chapter—children checking their alarm clocks once or twice on school nights—and superstitious behavior, both of which have no significant consequences, don't warrant a diagnosis of obsessive–compulsive disorder.)

Remember Camille, the little girl who is afraid someone is going to break into her home? Her nightly checking rituals go on so long that she ends up not getting enough sleep and is having trouble in school. Brenner, too, the child who was discussed at the start of this chapter, has rituals that are time-consuming. In his case they cause him to be late, creating a problem with sticking to his usual routine.

While compulsions themselves don't necessarily cause children to become distressed, kids *will* become extremely upset if they are blocked from performing them. For example, when six-year-old Asha's mom tried to keep her from arranging her stuffed animals, she threw a tantrum. Avery, a fourth grader with compulsive hand washing, threatened to run away from home when his dad prevented him from using the sink.

Kids get extremely upset if stopped from doing their rituals.

Although only one is required for a diagnosis, most kids have both obsessions and compulsions. And when kids do have compulsions, it's very often more than one. It's also not unusual for children's rituals to change over time. When Harry was little, he had a compulsion with arranging things. Now in fourth grade, he no longer does this, but he's developed a new problem—washing.

The Many Faces of Obsessive–Compulsive Disorder

As you've just seen, there are a number of different ways that obsessive-compulsive disorder can appear. Some children have both obsessions and compulsions, while others have just rituals. Also, the content of obsessions, as well as their intensity, frequency, and duration, varies. Compulsions, too, come in many forms, and the effects they have on children's lives are different.

With this in mind, let's now take an in-depth look at four children who have this disorder.

Kelly

Ten-year-old Kelly is obsessed with germs. She's panic-stricken if she comes into contact with someone who is, or later becomes, sick. She won't touch any of her friends' pets because she thinks animals are major carriers of disease. Kelly insists on wearing tops with sleeves that are too long so her hands are covered with fabric. That way she doesn't have to directly touch things that have been touched by a lot of other people, like the doorknob to the girls' room or the faucets on the bathroom sink at school.

Recently Kelly began to believe that her younger brother has "cooties" and is a source of contamination. She doesn't want to sit anywhere he's sat—in the car, at the kitchen table, on the sofa—or touch things he's touched and won't let him come into her room. She's even asked her mother to wash her clothes separately from his.

Kelly washes her hands so many times a day they've become red and scaly. When her friends ask her what's wrong, she says she has a skin problem. In fact her mom has taken her to see a dermatologist, but the doctor says there's really nothing he can do if she keeps on washing so much.

There's no doubt that Kelly has obsessive–compulsive disorder. She has obsessive thoughts about germs and tries to avoid coming into contact with them by covering her hands with fabric and staying away from animals, people with illnesses, and, unfortunately, her brother. She also excessively washes her hands, another compulsion that's common among kids with contamination fears.

Avoidance and washing rituals are common in kids who have contamination obsessions.

Kelly's obsession causes her a lot of distress, and her compulsions— particularly the avoidance rituals— keep her from doing things and going places that are normal for kids her age. Her singling out her brother as a source of contamination (not unusual for kids with contamination obsessions, although which family member is "selected" varies) also is creating tremendous stress and conflict at home. Moreover, it's starting to affect her brother's self-esteem—he's beginning to think maybe there *is* something wrong with him.

Omar

Omar, age eight, is preoccupied with how things are arranged. He makes sure all of the shoes in his closet are facing forward, lined up straight, and the same distance from each other. He also has a special way of arranging his toy cars and gets very upset if his mom accidentally moves any of them when she's straightening up his room.

Omar also lines up his feet so they're perfectly straight, while at the same time reciting silently in his head a list of seven things he

Kids Who Wash Too Much

Washing is the most common ritual of obsessive–compulsive children. As in Kelly's case, it can take the form of excessive hand washing. For other kids it involves frequent, elaborate (performed according to certain rules), or lengthy bathing or showering. Washing rituals often are triggered by obsessions about germs, illness, dirt, bodily excretions (mucus, urine, feces, saliva), or contamination from toxins in the environment.

likes to do. He has to say all seven activities in a specific order each time he goes through the list, and if he messes up he has to start over again. Omar also lines up his feet before he gets on his skateboard— he's always anxious about how he's going to do and thinks it will help him perform his tricks better.

It takes Omar at least ten minutes every morning to get his sneaker laces precisely the way he wants. If his dad interrupts him before he's done, pushing him to get going so he won't be late for school, he yells, "I won't go if my sneakers aren't right!"

It's clear that Omar has arranging and symmetry rituals that are time-consuming and also interfere with his normal routine. Reciting his list of activities meets the definition of a compulsion too, even though he does this mentally. Unlike Kelly, Omar isn't able to identify any clear-cut obsessive thoughts—he just feels compelled to perform his rituals, often when he's feeling anxious.

There's a bit of a "magical" quality to some of Omar's compulsions, like believing that lining up his feet will somehow make him do well at skateboarding. Compulsions that are performed in response to obsessions usually are intended to undo or prevent something bad from happening, as in Kelly's case. But when compulsions aren't linked to obsessions, as for Omar, they can be intended to make something good happen.

Even though he has several compulsions, Omar's friends don't know about them. Most of his rituals are done at home, so only his family sees them. Sometimes he lines up his feet when he's in class or playing with other kids, but so far he's been able to conceal this.

Holly

Twelve-year-old Holly has terrible thoughts. Blasphemous ideas keep entering her mind, like "I hate God" and even worse ones she feels she can't share with anybody. Coming from a religious family and going to parochial school, she feels incredibly guilty and can't understand why this is happening.

Holly also has another obsession. This one doesn't have to do with God, but it's just as bad. She has mental images of being raped. Holly has never been sexually assaulted and doesn't know anyone who has. In fact she hasn't had any kind of sexual experience yet, not even a kiss from a boy, so having images like these doesn't make any sense to her at all.

When Holly has one of her obsessions, she usually blinks really hard to get it to go away. Other times she tries to undo the bad thought by saying five Hail Marys in her head.

There's no question that Holly has obsessions. As we discussed earlier, thoughts and images with unacceptable religious and sexual content are two very common types of obsessions. Holly also has compulsions in response to her obsessions—blinking and praying, which are attempts to "neutralize" or undo the bad thing she has imagined.

Holly is experiencing a great deal of distress from her obsessions. Having sacrilegious and inappropriate sexual thoughts doesn't fit with Holly's self-concept. She feels guilty and bad about herself for having them. Although she's not clinically depressed at this time, she does have some symptoms of depression that may worsen if she doesn't get help for her problem soon.

Clarence

Clarence, a second grader, is showing some very strange behavior. He "redoes" things that don't need to be redone. For instance, he gets up from his chair, then immediately sits back down and then gets up again. He also walks back and forth through doorways and repeatedly flips light switches on and off.

Lately Clarence finds he often has to reread sentences, both when he's reading out loud and when he's reading silently to himself. His parents and teacher don't understand why—Clarence never had a problem with reading or reading comprehension before.

His mom has repeatedly asked him why he has to redo things, but Clarence has been reluctant to tell her. Finally he's admitted that he had been having thoughts that she is going to die. He thinks that in some way his repeating rituals will keep harm from coming her way.

Clarence's obsessive thoughts about his mother being harmed are triggering his redoing compulsions. As is true for many kids with obsessive–compulsive disorder, there's no logical connection between his obsessions and his rituals—repeating his actions can't prevent his mom from dying. Despite this, Clarence is compelled to do them. In fact, when his dad tries to physically stop him from re-doing something, Clarence becomes hysterical because he's certain something bad will happen to his mom.

Clarence has a form of obsessive–compulsive disorder that's very hard to hide. The bizarre appearance of his behavior causes other kids to tease him or stay away from him. His repeating rituals also are affecting his schoolwork—having to reread things makes doing his homework very time-consuming, and he often doesn't finish his assignments in class.

Getting Control of Obsessive–Compulsive Disorder

There are many things parents can do to help children with their obsessions and compulsions. Some of these involve using psychological techniques—ones I'll share with you shortly—that are designed to reduce these symptoms. Numerous research studies have shown these methods to be very effective, and for many kids they're all that's needed to bring obsessive–compulsive disorder under control.

Facts about Obsessive–Compulsive Disorder

Although obsessive–compulsive disorder is not uncommon in elementary-school-age kids, it's more *rare* than other childhood anxiety disorders.

The disorder occurs *more often in boys,* and boys usually develop it at an earlier age than girls.

Many children with obsessive–compulsive disorder have *multiple rituals*, not just one.

The most common compulsion is *washing.*

The disorder tends to be *chronic,* but "waxes and wanes." Kids alternate between periods of minimal symptoms and times when they are greatly increased.

For other kids, though, the techniques won't be enough by them-selves. These children will need the added help that comes from medication. While I know that no parent relishes the idea of having his or her child take psychiatric drugs, for certain kids with this dis-order getting better just isn't possible without them.

How do you know if you should consider this option for your child? First, if you find that using the techniques here does not make a significant improvement in your son or daughter's condi-tion, it's quite possible that a combination approach—medication in addition to the techniques—is what's needed. Other things to con-sider are the age when your child first developed OCD and whether the disorder runs in your family. If your child started showing ob-sessions or compulsions at a very early age (before five), or if he or she has close biological relatives with OCD (especially if the family members have severe forms of the disorder that first began during childhood or adolescence), drug therapy may be right for your child. Finally, when OCD symptoms are so pervasive and disruptive that they destroy a child's ability to have anything close to a normal life, parents should seriously consider a medication evaluation. You have very little to lose and potentially a lot to gain by getting the opinion of a physician who is an expert in this area.

If your child does need to take medication, it's still very important to use the techniques for controlling obsessions and compulsions that I've included here. (If you're not comfortable doing this by yourself, you can get assistance from a cognitive-behavioral psychologist who has experience with obsessive–compulsive children.) Although med-ication can be of great help in treating OCD, studies have shown that it's much more effective when combined with methods like these.

There's one more thing I want to share with you, although it's a bit difficult, before we turn to the methods that will help con-trol your child's obsessions and compulsions. As I've said before, obsessive–compulsive disorder tends to be a chronic disorder, one that virtually never goes away without an intervention. But what I didn't say earlier, that I want to share with you now, is that there are some kids who—even with treatment—won't be *100 percent free* of symptoms. Although they will be *much, much better*, possibly even 95 percent free of symptoms, some signs of the disorder may persist.

If your son or daughter falls into this category, the goal for you and your child shouldn't be to keep trying to *completely* get rid of all signs of the disorder, but, rather, to continue to work at keeping symptoms—and their effect on your child's life—to a minimum.

1. Keep your child's stress level down.

There's no question that stress makes obsessive–compulsive disorder worse. When kids are overly stressed, it's much more difficult for them to use the resources they naturally possess to combat this disorder.

Obviously it's not possible for your child to avoid all forms of stress. The normal day-to-day aspects of life and growing up have inherent stresses that can't be completely eliminated. But there are other types of stressors—ones I've included in the questionnaire on the following page—that you may be able to do something about.

Your child also can benefit from using one of the relaxation techniques that I talked about in Chapters 4 and 5. These methods can help reduce reactions to stresses that kids end up having to encounter because they decrease physiological arousal and help keep your son or daughter's anxiety level low.

Deep breathing (see Chapter 4, pages 111–112), which, as you'll recall, is learning to breathe deeply from the diaphragm, can be used pretty much anytime and anyplace because it's virtually undetectable (no one will know your child is doing it) and it takes only minutes to do. Deep muscle relaxation (see Chapter 5, pages 138–140), on the other hand, which involves systematically tensing and then relaxing a number of different muscles in the body in a specified sequence, is best done at home and is more time-consuming than the breathing technique. Because of this, if you and your child decide to use this relaxation method, consider scheduling a time for your child to do it. Once daily after school usually works well.

Remember at the beginning of this chapter I said that obsessive–compulsive disorder tends to "wax and wane"? The factor that's most responsible for whether OCD gets worse (waxes) or gets better (wanes) is stress. Keeping your child's stress level down will help to keep his or her symptoms to a minimum. You and your child can then use the techniques for controlling obsessions and compulsions included in this section much more effectively.

2. Reduce the frequency of obsessions with the record-keeping approach.

As we've already seen, obsessions cause children a lot of distress and also, in most cases, lead to compulsions. Reducing the frequency of obsessions your child experiences will in turn reduce your child's discomfort and, if he or she does have compulsions, the time spent ritualizing.

> **Getting rid of obsessions also often improves compulsions.**

For many kids the record-keeping method works very well at decreasing the frequency of obsessions. This very simple procedure involves keeping track of obsessions as they're happening (or right after they happen) by recording their occurrence on paper.

The weekly record form on page 160 can be used to do this. When having an obsessive thought your child should go to the space that's been provided for that day and make a checkmark. This

---

Is Your Child Overly Stressed?

1. Are you pushing your child too hard to achieve—at school, in sports, or in any other activities?

2. Is your child's schedule too crowded? Does he or she have too many planned activities and not enough "downtime"?

3. Are conflicts in the family—such as problems between you and your child's other parent, if there is one—stressing your child?

4. Have any major changes recently occurred—like a move to a new house, the death of a pet, a serious illness in a family member?

5. Does your child get enough rest? Does he or she have too little sleep or poor-quality sleep? (If so, see Chapter 5, page 133, for how to improve this.)

6. Do you or your child's other parent have trouble managing your own stress? Do you have trouble keeping emotions under control when interacting with your child?

7. Does your child engage in a lot of overstimulating activities—ones that put him or her on edge?

should be done *every* time your child has the obsession, so if he or she has them very frequently there may (at least at first) be a lot of checkmarks crowded into the space. (If there isn't enough room because your child's obsessions occur so often, a separate piece of paper can be used for each day of the week instead of the form.)

I want to emphasize that for this technique to work it's very important that children record their obsessions either while they are occurring or *right* afterward, not later on. That means your child will need to keep the form (or piece of paper) and a pencil readily available as much of the time as possible. (Obviously there are certain activities your child will be involved in where it just won't be possible to have these things nearby or to fill out the form right away.) Extra copies of the form are at the back of the book.

You will know the technique is working when you see the number of checkmarks decreasing. You can total the number of checkmarks for each day and look for this trend, but sometimes improvement is better measured by using weekly averages—just add up the total number of checkmarks for a week and divide by seven.

Ten-year-old Maggie has an obsession about dirt. The first week she kept her record she and her mom discovered that she was troubled by these thoughts an average of fifteen times a day. During the second week of record keeping the average went down to ten, and by the end of the third week it was four. After a couple more weeks of using this method she hardly had any obsessive thoughts at all.

Although the technique can be used by kids of almost any age, younger children may find it difficult to do their record keeping without drawing attention to themselves. While you don't want your child to feel ashamed about the obsessions, it's probably best that other kids remain unaware that your child has them (as you know, kids aren't always kind about other children's problems). When children aren't able to do the record keeping in a way that stays private, I recommend they do it only when they are with their families or by themselves. While this isn't the very best way to use this method, it's a compromise that still works for many kids.

While this happens *very rarely*, I want to mention that it's possible for children to become more distressed from their obsessions when they start recording them or to develop rituals over completing the form. For example, Josh, a fourth grader, keeps having doubts about

Weekly Record

Monday

_____

_____

Tuesday

_____

_____

Wednesday

_____

_____

Thursday

_____

_____

Friday

_____

_____

Saturday

_____

_____

Sunday

_____

_____

whether he made checkmarks when he was supposed to. He spends a lot of time checking and rechecking his form.

Although, as I said, responses like Josh's happen infrequently, there's no way of predicting which children will have them. If your child develops a problem like this, please discontinue using this method and move on to the other ones I've included in this section.

Although several theories have been proposed, researchers really aren't sure why the act of recording one's own symptoms ends up reducing them. As a parent of a child with OCD, though, you probably find it less important to understand why the technique works than to know that it does.

3. Take the distress out of your child's obsession.

Many children, and adults too for that matter, have strange, unsettling thoughts that really don't make sense. For the most part, thoughts like these don't become obsessions. But when they do it's largely because of the intense negative emotions they trigger (if the thoughts just went in and out of your child's head without a major emotional reaction, they wouldn't become obsessions).

Reducing the distress that obsessions cause is an important component to getting rid of them and, if your child has compulsions too, the rituals they fuel. "Overexposing" children to their disturbing thoughts or images is an approach that gets rid of this emotional reaction. The procedure essentially involves kids repeatedly having their obsessions for an extended period of time without trying to suppress them or engaging in any compulsions (mental or behavioral) in response to them. Through this process the emotional aspect of obsessions eventually dissipates, and when the obsession no longer triggers discomfort or distress, it occurs less frequently, often going away completely.

There are several different ways that overexposure can be done, but I'll be sharing with you the method that I use, the one I have found works best with children. With this method kids intentionally try to produce their obsessive thoughts or images nonstop for periods ranging from five to fifteen minutes (five or ten minutes for younger kids, fifteen minutes for older children). (In contrast to this approach, children's obsessions can be presented to them—for instance, by a therapist—rather than having kids bring them on themselves. But I prefer that only professionals, not parents, use this method in this way.)

To use this technique you and your child will first need to pick a time and place where the overexposure sessions will be conducted. It's important that the same time and place be used for each session. The place should be quiet, and your child should be able to lie down, as in the child's bedroom. When choosing a time it's probably best to stay away from bedtime or right before school. Before or after dinner usually works well. Also, your child will need a timer that's easy for him or her to operate (a kitchen-style, portable timer—like an egg timer—is good), which can be set for up to fifteen minutes and has a ringer or other noise that's loud enough to alert your child that an overexposure session is finished.

Tell your child that the two of you are going to be working on a way to make the obsession less upsetting—in fact, you're going to be making it "boring." Explain—in a way that's appropriate to your child's age—that having the obsessive thought (or mental picture) over and over again for a pretty long period of time will eventually make it seem like it's not so bad or disturbing anymore.

Once all of this is in place, you're ready to begin. Have your child set the timer for the length of the overexposure period and then lie down with eyes closed. For the next five (or ten or fifteen) minutes your child is to say the obsessive thought repeatedly, silently in his or her head, until the ringer goes off. If your child's obsession is a mental image, the picture should be brought into his or her head and then kept there and focused on for the entire time period. Kids may find they lose their concentration during overexposure sessions, but let them know that it's very important that they keep the obsessive thought (or image) in their minds the whole time. If they drift off and daydream, they need to catch themselves and get back to focusing on the obsession right away.

It is absolutely critical that children do not try to actively suppress the obsession during the overexposure session or respond to it—trying to counteract, undo, or "neutralize" it—with mental rituals or compulsive behaviors. To make sure this problem doesn't arise with your child, you need to know how your child typically responds to his or her obsession so you can emphasize what should *not* be done during the overexposure session. Let's see how Nadine's mom dealt with this issue.

Nadine is a ten-year-old with a very disturbing obsession that she doesn't understand. From five to ten times a day the thought "I'm going to kill my mom with a knife" comes into her mind. For a long time Nadine didn't share what she regarded as "her secret" with her mother because she was so ashamed. But her mom suspected something was wrong anyway—periodically she would see a really "spooked" look come across her daughter's face, and then Nadine would start humming. The humming would go on for anywhere from a few seconds to a few minutes.

After much questioning Nadine finally told her mom about the thoughts. They decided to use the overexposure method to try to get rid of them, but after several weeks they didn't seem to be getting anywhere. Finally, one day, purely by accident, Nadine's mom happened to pass by her daughter's bedroom while she was doing her overexposure session and heard Nadine humming. From reading this chapter Nadine's mother suspected that the humming probably was a compulsion that was being used to "counteract" the obsessive thought.

After her discovery, Nadine's mom told her daughter to try her very, very hardest not to hum during the overexposure sessions. After two weeks of using the procedure—without the humming—Nadine's obsession was gone.

Overexposure sessions should be done once every day for at least two weeks. Two weeks usually is long enough to extinguish the negative emotions associated with an obsession. When this happens, the obsession will occur much less frequently or even, like for Nadine, not at all. If your child is using the record-keeping approach (see technique 1, above) while doing the overexposure, which I recommend, it will let you know this is occurring.

I want to mention that some kids, even when they try their hardest, find they aren't able to bring on their obsessions or can do it for only a very brief amount of time. Although these children really aren't doing overexposure, so in theory they shouldn't be getting better, in many cases their obsessions disappear anyway. This type of reaction is not uncommon when using this particular form of overexposure, and when it happens it's through a different process from the one I discussed earlier (the obsession goes away not because the negative emotions attached to it disappear, but through a process called *paradoxical intention*), but the positive effects are just as lasting.

One of the reasons I prefer this particular method of over-exposure among its many variations is because of the possibility of kids improving in this way. In addition, most kids find the idea of controlling their own overexposure—as opposed to having someone else, like a parent or therapist, be in charge of it—less scary. As a result they're usually more receptive to doing it.

4. Help your child learn how to cut obsessing time short.

Eleven-year-old Donald is obsessed with the idea of death. He can't stop thinking about how it feels to die and what will happen to him after he dies. Sometimes the thoughts go on for a really long time and he misses out on what's going on around him. Last night during his favorite TV show, for example, he was obsessing the whole time it was on.

Some children have obsessions that are fleeting, just lasting for a few seconds, while others kids—like Donald—have ones that go on much longer, for many minutes or even hours. When the duration of obsessions is a problem, the *thought-stopping* procedure should be used.

> When obsessions go on for many minutes or hours, thought stopping is the technique to use.

The idea behind this technique is to cut off obsessions as close to their onset as possible so they end up going on for a much shorter period of time. How is this done? Children simply shout the word "STOP!" as loud as they can as soon as they catch themselves beginning to obsess. If kids are in a place where they should not shout out loud, like around people other than their families, they can either whisper "stop!" under their breath or "yell" the word in their heads without saying anything out loud.

A frequently used variant of the original thought-stopping procedure is for children to close their eyes and imagine a pleasant scene right after they've interrupted their obsession with "stop." To really be effective, pleasant scenes should be based on kids' own personal experiences and preferences. For example, Chloe, a third grader, likes to picture herself at her family's summer home. After stopping his obsession, nine-year-old Damien imagines himself playing basketball.

Although the addition of the pleasant scene seems to work well for many kids, it's not always feasible to do because it requires children to close their eyes. There's another elaboration of the thought-stopping technique, though, that doesn't have this drawback. It involves applying a mildly uncomfortable physical stimulus in addition to saying the word "stop." A rubber band "snap" often is used for this.

Children wear some kind of elasticized or stretchy band (make sure it's not too tight) on one of their wrists—on the left wrist if right-handed, on the right wrist if left-handed—all of the time, except while sleeping. (Later on, after kids get their obsessions under pretty good control, wearing the band can be discontinued and they can just use the word *stop*.) The band can be a common rubber band that's found in any office supply store. Girls often prefer to wear a hair accessory on their wrists, like a ponytail holder or a scrunchie, instead of a rubber band. There also are unisex bracelets that have stretchy cords (you usually can find these at a kiosk at the mall) that both boys and girls can use.

To use this method of thought stopping children cut their obsessions short with "stop" as described earlier, but *at the same time* they pull the band away from their wrists so that when it retracts it causes a mild stinging sensation.

Although research suggests that adding the rubber band makes the thought-stopping procedure more effective, some kids—particularly younger ones—have trouble doing it without drawing attention to themselves (which you definitely don't want). Also, some parents just aren't comfortable with the idea of their children "hurting" themselves, even though the sensation from the rubber band is very, very mild.

From my experience, the addition of the rubber band really does make a big difference, so I'm in favor of doing thought stopping this way. Hopefully, when you weigh the very minor physical discomfort the band may cause against its potential benefits, you'll come to the same conclusion. But if you don't, still go ahead and have your child use one of the other thought-stopping methods discussed earlier. Even without the rubber band it will be very helpful in reducing the time your child spends obsessing.

To get the most out of the thought-stopping procedure—regardless of which particular method is used—children need to catch themselves and use the technique *every time* they're obsessing. It's not unusual for kids at first to have to repeat the procedure several times to get an obsession to leave and *stay* away. Eventually, though, this won't be the case—a single "stop" will be all it takes.

Before leaving this topic I want to remind you that the thought-stopping procedure is not for all kids who have obsessions. It's only for kids who spend lengthy periods at a time obsessing, not for kids who have brief, fleeting obsessive thoughts or images.

If your child is an appropriate candidate for the thought-stopping procedure, he or she also can use the other methods for dealing with obsessions that I talked about earlier. However, depending on other aspects of your child's obsession, record keeping and overexposure may or may not be as helpful as the thought-stopping approach. Record keeping usually makes the biggest impact on obsessions where frequency—not duration—is the main problem, while overexposure works best for obsessions that trigger major emotional reactions.

If your child's situation suggests he or she may benefit from the other methods, go ahead and use them. I would recommend, though, that you not have your child do all three at the same time. Start off with the thought-stopping procedure alone or a combination of record keeping and overexposure. If after a period of time

Which Methods Are Right for Your Child?

Record keeping	For *frequent* obsessions
Overexposure	When obsessions trigger a lot of *distress*
Thought stopping	For *lengthy* obsessions

you're not completely satisfied with how your child is doing, switch to the other method (or methods) for handling obsessions.

Ten-year-old Julio started by using the record-keeping approach and having daily overexposure sessions. After a couple of weeks his obsessions were less frequent and not as distressing, but when they did occur they would go on for fifteen or twenty minutes at a time. He started using the thought-stopping technique, and his time spent obsessing decreased dramatically. Ultimately for Julio, as for many other kids who have obsessions, all three techniques played a role in getting better.

5. Avoid feeding into your child's compulsions

Kids usually are pretty good about working on their obsessions. Because they are so upsetting and disturbing, they *want* to get rid of them. But compulsions typically don't cause anxiety and distress as obsessions do. In fact it's usually the opposite—they reduce discomfort. Also, as you'll recall from our discussion earlier, most children don't recognize that their compulsive behavior is excessive or irrational—it's parents who identify the rituals as a problem.

For these reasons children are very motivated to *keep* doing their rituals. And to make sure they're able to do so they frequently get their families—especially their parents, but sometimes brothers and sisters too—to do things that make it easier for them to perform their compulsions.

Enabling kids to perform their compulsions is always the wrong move. At the time it might seem like the right thing to do because its immediate effect is to reduce your child's anxiety and distress. But because compulsions reduce anxiety, they are self-reinforcing, so allowing children to ritualize actually ends up making their OCD worse.

Do you remember Kelly, the girl who refused to be in contact with anything her brother touched because she believed he had "cooties"? Thinking they were helping her, Kelly's parents made it possible for her to avoid the situations that made her anxious. For example, they let her sit in the front seat of the car, where her brother never sat, while her mom rode in the back. And they agreed—at Kelly's insistence—that her brother would never be allowed on "Kelly's side" of the family room sofa.

What could Kelly's folks have done differently? The best thing would have been to say "No!" to her attempts at avoidance. Doing this, though, wouldn't have been easy. Kelly's anxiety probably would have skyrocketed when her parents refused to give in to her demands. She even might have had a panic attack, thrown a tantrum, or threatened her folks. But eventually her anxiety and distress would have subsided, and then her urges to avoid her brother would have decreased too. By being blocked from doing her avoidance rituals Kelly would have begun to get better.

Like Kelly, nine-year-old Tatiana has a parent who is making special accommodations because of her daughter's OCD. Tatiana has an obsession with dirt and germs. She refuses to use a towel or wear a piece of clothing more than once without having it washed. Since she's too young to do the laundry herself, this places tremendous demands on her mom, who, in an effort to keep Tatiana from getting upset, has taken on the job.

It definitely would have been better for Tatiana if her mom had not made things so easy for her. Being forced to reuse a towel and wear clothing more than once (assuming it really isn't dirty) would have helped Tatiana get past her problem.

As another example, let's look at Elliot and his dad. Elliot is a sixth grader who has an obsession that his home is going to be destroyed in a fire. He spends a lot of time repeatedly checking things he believes could cause a fire—for example, that the range and stove are turned off, that his mom's electric curlers are unplugged, and that the lighter for the barbecue has the safety latch on. But no matter how many times Elliot checks and rechecks, he's always afraid that he's missed something or not done one of the rituals "completely" or "right." He wants his dad to go through them with him so he can feel more secure.

It's easy to understand why Elliot's father agreed to watch his son go through his rituals. He thought he was helping his child. But although having Dad "double-check" his compulsions gave Elliot some immediate relief, in the long run it prolonged his OCD. Providing reassurance—through double-checking or in another way I'll discuss next—strengthens kids' compulsions and any obsessions attached to them because it reduces anxiety. (What should Elliot's dad have done instead? See strategy 6, below.)

Parents also can provide reassurance, and inadvertently feed into their children's compulsions, by responding to OCD-related questions. We already talked about how to handle requests for reassurance in the last chapter with regard to generalized anxiety disorder. For OCD the same basic procedure is used.

Let's go back to Kelly for a minute, the girl who avoids contact with her brother. To be certain she hasn't accidentally touched anything of his, she bombards her mom with questions about her and her brother's behavior. For instance, during dinner she asks, "Did I brush up against Ryan when I came into the kitchen?" "Did Ryan touch my chair?" "Did he touch my dinner plate?" and so on.

Besides being annoying to listen to, and making her brother feel bad, Kelly's requests for reassurance are problematic in another way. If her mom answers the questions and gives her daughter the reassurance she seeks, Kelly's anxiety, for the moment, will lessen. But just as for Elliot, the anxiety reduction then will make her compulsions (and the obsessions related to them) even stronger.

How, then, should Kelly's mom respond to her questions? In one of two ways—by either saying "You know I can't answer that (because it will make your problem worse)"

> **Reassuring children on OCD-related issues isn't helpful.**
>
> **It actually makes the disorder worse.**

or by completely ignoring them. Obviously she should tell her child about the new way she will be handling questions before she begins to do so. It's also important that she explain to Kelly why she's taking on this approach (for example, "to help you with your problem"), so that mom's change in behavior isn't interpreted as a form of rejection.

I know that not responding to requests for reassurance may sound like—and feel like—an insensitive thing to do to your distressed child. It's important to remember, though, that by answering OCD-related questions you really aren't helping your child. As I said before, providing reassurance in this way actually makes your child's condition worse.

When you start dealing with your child's reassurance seeking in either of the ways I suggest, you may find, at first, that there's an escalation in anxiety, possibly resulting in the type of reactions I talked about earlier (tantrums, panic attacks, threats). Be assured that this will go away soon, as long as you stick with your new approach. You also may find that your child keeps repeating the same question many times in an effort to get you to respond, but when this doesn't work (make sure you don't respond!), this behavior will stop too.

6. Help your child get rid of compulsions by reducing the urge to ritualize.

While it's very important for parents not to enable or feed into their children's compulsions by making special provisions for them or responding to reassurance-seeking questions, doing this alone won't be enough to get compulsions under control. Parents also need methods that help stop their children from doing their rituals when they have urges to perform them.

Consider eleven-year-old Patrick's situation. Patrick is a compulsive hand washer. Although, after reading this chapter, his mom no longer goes along with his OCD-related requests, Patrick still washes his hands far more than is normal. What should Patrick's mom do when he goes to wash?

Urges to engage in a compulsion dissipate over time. Given that this is the case, if Patrick's mom can get her son to agree to hold off on doing the washing by waiting for a certain period of time, chances are that when the time period is over he no longer will feel the need to perform his ritual. How long should she ask Patrick to wait? Generally, the longer the period of time, the more likely the

Postponing a ritual lessens the urge to perform it.

method is to be effective (that's because with more time there's a better chance the urge will have passed). However, Patrick's mother may find she has to negotiate with her son the length of the delay to get him to agree to it.

When Patrick's mom suggested that he wait a half hour and then see if he still needed to wash, Patrick insisted it be for only five minutes. His mom then came back with a compromise of fifteen minutes, which Patrick finally agreed to. (If you have difficulty getting your child to agree to postpone the compulsion for *any* length of time, try using small rewards as incentives. See Chapter 4, pages 112–113, for how to go about doing this.)

What do you do if your child still has the urge to perform the compulsion at the end of the delay period? Negotiate for an additional delay. Sometimes the initial period of time isn't long enough for the urge to go away completely, but lengthening the time with another delay does the trick.

The delay technique is a great tool for helping kids get rid of urges to perform compulsions. But sometimes using it isn't feasible—such as at school, because you're not there, or in other instances where you don't know exactly when your child's rituals are occurring, or if your child's rituals are so pervasive that using the technique would mean that he or she would be in an almost perpetual state of "delay."

In these cases for children to overcome their compulsions parents will need to take a more aggressive approach, one that involves actively implementing measures that prevent or interfere with kids' carrying out their rituals. This approach to dealing with compulsions is known as *response prevention*. When kids are blocked from performing their compulsions (preventing the "response"), the urge to do them will eventually go away. Let's look at Patrick again—the compulsive hand washer—so you can see response prevention in action.

The delay technique was helpful for cutting back on some of Patrick's washing at home. But his mom suspects that Patrick may be washing excessively at school because his teacher told her that he asks to go the restroom a lot. Also, Patrick's mother is pretty sure he's still washing at home at times she doesn't know about. For instance, if she's in the kitchen—on the first floor—Patrick could easily be washing upstairs and she'd be unaware of it.

> **Urges to perform their compulsions go away when kids are blocked from performing them.**

Patrick's mom decided to use response prevention—both at school and at home—to get Patrick's washing under control. To stop her son from washing too much at school she asked his teacher not to give Patrick permission to go to the restroom so often, to limit him to one time in the morning and one time in the afternoon. She also was able to arrange for one of the school's guidance counselors (a male) to accompany her son on trips to the bathroom to make sure he wasn't "overwashing" (spending more than a minute washing) at these times.

Patrick also was blocked from excessively washing at home. His parents had most of the faucets in their home disabled, except in places where they would be able to exert control over Patrick's behavior (the bathroom in his parents' master bedroom suite—because it's a place not readily accessible to him—and in the kitchen, which is a "high traffic" area where his family would see him if he attempted to use the sink to wash).

I'm sure that some of you who are reading this probably think it was pretty extreme of Patrick's parents to shut off the faucets in their home. At a minimum I'm certain it was very inconvenient for all the members of Patrick's family. But for a child who has frequent compulsions it's often necessary to go to lengths like these to get rid of the behavior. (I also should point out that the changes Patrick's parents made to their home were only temporary. Once Patrick's hand washing was under control the faucets were turned back on.)

Getting Patrick into a normal pattern of hand washing made his urges to wash excessively go away. Was this easy to accomplish? No. It took considerable effort on the part of his school and his family over a period of a couple of months. But the reward was well worth the time and effort spent (and the inconvenience too). Today, one year later, Patrick still has his washing under control.

Sometimes using response prevention entails being pretty creative, which is what happened with my eight-year-old patient Omar, introduced earlier in this chapter. To refresh your memory, Omar is the boy who spends a lot of time arranging and lining up things, like the shoes in his closet and his toy cars.

When Omar puts his shoes on the floor of his closet, it gets him started on arranging them. So to deal with the shoe problem I suggested to Omar and his mom that they adopt a completely different approach to putting shoes away. I asked Omar's mom to tack a carpet remnant on the back wall of her son's closet. From now on, instead of placing his shoes on the floor of his closet—the behavior that gets him started on arranging them—Omar was instructed to throw his shoes against the carpet on the back wall, just letting them land where they may. (By the way, Omar responded very enthusiastically to this idea—he thought "the game" would be a lot of fun.)

When Omar and his mother came back the next week, they reported that shoes no longer were an issue. Omar was pitching them into the closet and living with them, quite comfortably, in disarray.

In this case using response prevention—preventing the "response" (the compulsion)—involved coming up with an alternative behavior, one that made doing the ritualized behavior impossible. You'll remember that when I first mentioned response prevention to you I said that it either interfered with or prevented kids from doing their rituals. Here, for Omar's shoes, the throwing of them *interfered* with, or competed with, his arranging ritual—he couldn't toss them into disarray and arrange them at the same time. (If Omar had gotten into arranging his shoes after scattering them, which he did not, I would have handled his shoe compulsion much like Patrick's hand washing—*preventing* Omar from arranging shoes in his closet by keeping him locked out of it.)

The next thing to tackle was Omar's compulsion with his toy cars. Response prevention also was used to get this problem under control, but here we included an *exposure* component as part of the procedure. This involved having Omar see his cars "out of order" and not be allowed to put them back "in order."

I told Omar's mom to begin by *slightly* altering Omar's arrangement of his cars and then not letting him rearrange them. To get Omar through this she used the delay technique that I talked about earlier. As would be expected, Omar was somewhat distressed at first at seeing his cars "messed up," but as the delay period went on his discomfort with the situation subsided, and after about ten minutes he no longer had urges to put them back in order. This exercise was repeated several times, till it was clear that Omar no longer had any difficulty with it.

Next I asked Omar's mom to make the situation just a little more difficult, this time altering the arrangement of the cars in a way that was slightly more askew than before and again using the delay technique. It took a longer delay period and more repetitions for Omar to finally be okay with this step, but eventually he was able to tolerate his cars being like this.

Omar's mom continued the exposure and response prevention exercises in this way, slowly increasing the difficulty of the steps over a period of eight weeks. By the end of the two months she had Omar's cars scattered all over his room, not at all resembling the carefully constructed order he used to keep them in. Now Omar continues to enjoy playing with his cars much in the way many other little boys do, no longer having the urge to arrange them.

If, like Omar, your child has a compulsion that can be approached by using exposure along with response prevention, break things down into small steps and begin with an exposure that will cause only a minimal amount of anxiety. Once a step has been "mastered" (it no longer is hard to do) you can proceed to a more difficult one, but make sure it's only slightly harder than the one before it. If you mistakenly ask your child to do a step that's too much of a jump (in terms of its difficulty), the delay technique won't work and you'll have quite a battle on your hands. Remember, the object of response prevention is for your child *not* to perform his or her ritual. To make sure this happens you're far better off coming up with steps that are too easy than taking the risk that they will be too hard.

As you know from reading this chapter, there are many things families can do to help children who have OCD. I've included several techniques that you can teach your child that can get rid of obsessive thoughts and shown you how to approach—and eliminate—your child's compulsive behavior. With this information you now have a variety of tools you can use to bring your child's obsessions and compulsions under control. But remember, if these strategies aren't of significant help to your child, it's wise to see a mental health professional, either for help with these or similar techniques or to arrange for a medication evaluation.

7 SELF-CONSCIOUS TO A FAULT
Social Anxiety Disorder

Ashton has always been shy, but since her family moved she's been much worse. She's been in her new school now for over four months but still hardly talks to any of the kids. She doesn't participate in the group games at recess, instead standing off to the side by herself. During lunch she eats alone and keeps her head down to avoid making eye contact with her classmates.

Ashton never raises her hand when the teacher asks a question or initiates one of her own. She doesn't like having attention drawn to her because she's afraid she'll look or sound stupid. She's not only worried about what the other kids will think; she's overly concerned about her teacher's opinion too.

When she's with her family or visits with her friends from her old neighborhood, Ashton is just like her old self. How can she bring her "old self" into her new environment? Is there anything her parents or teacher can do to help?

As we discussed at the very beginning of this book, all kids go through a period when they're uncomfortable around people they don't know well. "Stranger anxiety," as it's often called, usually makes its first appearance between the ages of one and two and then goes away by around two and a half years. Some children continue to exhibit signs of shyness after this time, but when they begin school and spend more time with other kids this usually goes away.

In some cases, though, increased social interactions don't help children become more comfortable. Instead their shyness intensifies and becomes more of a problem, causing kids a lot of distress and interfering with their ability to function in social settings. When this happens, the possibility of social anxiety disorder should be considered.

Although shyness often is a precursor to social anxiety disorder, the two differ in many ways. Shy children usually have friends, while socially anxious children often have none, or only one or two. Shy children may be reluctant to enter certain social situations but rarely avoid them, while the opposite is true of kids with social anxiety disorder. Shy children often are uncomfortable—at least initially—in some social settings, but they don't experience the level of intense physiological arousal (such as, for example, panic attacks) and distress that is characteristic of social anxiety disorder. Finally, shy children basically are able to live relatively normal lives. Kids with social anxiety disorder, on the other hand, don't. They're unable to do many of the things that other kids their age do.

Social anxiety disorder does not go away on its own. In fact, not only does it continue, but it usually gets worse as kids get older, particularly when they are adolescents and young adults. Teens with social anxiety disorder not only are limited in their friendships; they're extremely uncomfortable interacting with the opposite sex (this might sound good to you at first, but believe me, it really is a problem!). They don't date, don't go to school dances, and don't go to the prom, leaving them feeling isolated and like they don't fit in, which, in some cases, can lead to depression. When the time comes for college, they often are afraid to go away to school, instead opting to attend a local community college and continuing to live at home, as found in a study we reported in a 1998 article in the *Journal of the American Academy of Child and Adolescent Psychiatry*. As young adults they're frequently limited in their potential for career advancement because they are timid and anxious around their superiors.

If your child has social anxiety disorder, his or her future does not have to be restricted in this way. There are many things the two of you can do right now to help your child overcome this problem. But before we get to that, let's look at this anxiety disorder in more depth and see whether the description really fits your child.

Diagnosing Social Anxiety Disorder

As you can see in the sidebar below, the hallmark of social anxiety disorder, or *social phobia* as it also is referred to, is a severe fear of a social or performance situation because of excessive concern about acting or looking in a way that will be humiliating or embarrassing.

> The real fear of socially anxious children is of being publicly embarrassed or humiliated.

Social anxiety disorder comes in two forms. The first form is the *generalized* type. Children with generalized social phobia are extremely anxious in most social situations. They have great difficulty interacting with children their age, but they also can have problems with older or younger children and adults. Children with generalized social phobia have difficulty initiating and maintaining conversations with other kids, tend to "shrink" from contact with them (often preferring to stay close to familiar adults), are very uncomfortable in groups of children and may refuse to participate in group play (instead choosing to stay on the "sidelines"), and may be anxious speaking to authority figures

Symptoms of Social Anxiety Disorder

To be diagnosed with this disorder, a child must have these symptoms:

- Is extremely fearful of at least one situation involving social contact or requiring some kind of performance, where the child will be exposed to or scrutinized by unfamiliar children (not just adults).
- Fears that he or she will act or look in a way that will be humiliating or embarrassing.
- Either avoids the feared situation(s) or experiences severe anxiety or distress when in the situation(s).
- Either has his or her normal routine, schoolwork, social activities, or relationships disrupted by the phobia or is extremely distressed about having the phobia.
- Has experienced this fear for at least six months.

Children with the generalized form of social phobia are anxious in almost all social situations.

like their teachers. Ashton, the girl introduced at the beginning of this chapter, is a good example of a child who has this problem.

The other form of social phobia is the *circumscribed* type. Here the situations that make children uncomfortable are more specific or limited. Circumscribed social phobias can focus on either social or performance situations. Some common ones include fears of speaking or performing in front of others, eating in public, being in crowded places, blushing, using public restrooms, and undressing in front of other (same-sex) children. Let's look at a few examples:

- Imani, like many other preteen girls, is preoccupied with her appearance. But unlike most kids her age, she's extremely uncomfortable being in large groups or crowded situations because she thinks people are looking at her and seeing her faults.
- Nine-year-old Marcus doesn't want to use the bathroom at school unless there are no other kids in the room. He's embarrassed by the sounds he makes when he does "number two."
- Alexandra, age ten, has "developed" early and is the only girl in her class who wears a bra. She is extremely uncomfortable changing into her gym clothes in front of the other girls and tries to stay home from school on days that she has phys ed.
- Wiley is a seven-year-old who is very fair skinned and blushes easily. Having been teased by kids about this, he frequently checks his face in the mirror for any sign of redness, anxious and worried that it will happen and he'll be embarrassed again.

Excessive fears about vomiting also are very common in children, but they can be diagnosed as either a social or a specific phobia, depending on what the child fears. It's diagnosed as a social phobia if the fear primarily is about the potential embarrassment of throwing up in front of others, as opposed to the physical act of vomiting itself (then it would be a specific phobia—see Chapter 8).

Regardless of whether kids have the generalized or circumscribed form of the disorder, children react to the situations they fear by trying to avoid them. Often they can't do this because their parents won't allow it. For instance, Alexandra (the girl I just spoke about who doesn't want to change her clothes for gym class) can't get her folks to let her to stay home from school no matter how hard she tries.

But some kids are successful at avoiding the situations they fear because the way they go about it is more subtle than flat out refusing to do something or go somewhere and not as easy for parents or others to detect. As examples of this, let's look at three children who all have social phobias about eating in front of others, each of whom has a different way of avoiding having lunch at school.

As a sixth grader, Ruth has the option of going home to have lunch, which she does every day. Audrey forgoes lunch entirely, waiting till she gets home from school to eat. Chelsea sits in the cafeteria during lunchtime and pretends to eat by playing with and picking at her food.

If children can't avoid the situations they fear, they endure them with intense anxiety or distress. Some children have panic attacks when forced to be in their feared situations. Others cry, throw tantrums, freeze, or "shrink" from the people around them.

Six-year-old Victor tries to hide behind furniture when he has to be around people he doesn't know. Karen, a sixth grader, has full-blown panic attacks—heart racing, hands trembling, hyperventilating—when she has to give a presentation at school. During her violin recital eight-year-old Melinda completely froze up and was unable to play.

To receive the diagnosis of social anxiety disorder your child must be extremely distressed about having the phobia, or the social or performance anxiety must interfere significantly with some aspect of functioning. For example, Marisol is so consumed with what the other students are thinking of her that she can't pay attention and her grades are suffering. Amber's social anxiety is so severe that she literally has to be *physically forced* to go to school. Lydia is so nervous around other kids that it's almost impossible for her to make friends.

Marisol, Amber, and Lydia all have the generalized type of social phobia. Usually children who have the generalized form of this disorder are more impaired than kids who have the circumscribed form because of the *sheer number* of situations that are difficult for them. (However, when children have two or more circumscribed social phobias—which, by the way, isn't at all unusual—the impact on their lives can become more akin to what kids with generalized social phobia experience.) Generalized social phobia can significantly interfere with all or almost all of your child's social interactions, affecting the ability to form relationships and participate in activities with others. In addition, it's very common for kids with generalized social anxiety disorder to have phobias of performance situations as well—like giving a presentation in front of the class, performing in a play, or giving a recital. Then the number of situations that are problematic for them increases even more.

The questionnaire on the facing page will help you pinpoint which particular social and performance situations are problematic for your child and also give you some idea of whether your child has the generalized or circumscribed form of social phobia. (The G or C that appears in parentheses at the end of each item tells you whether a fear of that situation is indicative of a generalized—G—or circumscribed—C—social phobia. A few of the items have both a G and C after them, which means they can occur in both forms of the disorder.) This information will be particularly important when we get to some of the strategies you and your child will use to overcome social anxiety disorder. It also will help you to see where your child's situation lies, which will be particularly helpful as we now take an in-depth look at some kids who already have been diagnosed with social anxiety disorder.

The Many Faces of Social Anxiety Disorder

As you've just seen, social anxiety disorder can appear in a number of different ways. Some kids have the generalized form of the disorder, affecting all, or almost all, social situations, while other kids have the circumscribed form of the disorder, affecting a more limited number of circumstances. Some social phobias have to do solely with social interactions, while others target just performance situations, and yet still others affect both types of situations.

The Social Anxiety Questionnaire

Is your child. . .	Yes	No
1. Excessively concerned about looking stupid, foolish, or incompetent or about being embarrassed? Worried about not "acting right" or "looking right"? (G, C)	☐	☐
2. Uncomfortable eating or drinking in front of others except for family or very close friends? (C)	☐	☐
3. Extremely uncomfortable giving (or unable to give) oral reports or presentations in front of the class? (G, C)	☐	☐
4. Resistant to ever raising his or her hand to ask or answer a question at school? (G)	☐	☐
5. Very uncomfortable being the center of attention? (G, C)	☐	☐
6. Unable to talk to children he or she doesn't know (or very uncomfortable doing so)? (G)	☐	☐
7. Without close friends (or has only one or two)? (G)	☐	☐
8. Avoidant of or extremely uncomfortable in situations where changing clothing in front of others is required—such as at gym class, swimming practice, ballet, or camp? (C)	☐	☐
9. Very reluctant to have children come over to the house for a play date, sleepover, or birthday party? (G)	☐	☐
10. Persistently worried about the possibility of blushing in front of others? (C)	☐	☐
11. Unable to use public restrooms unless no one else is in them? (C)	☐	☐
12. Extremely anxious or unable to perform in front of others—like in a recital, play, or sports event? (C)	☐	☐
13. Very anxious in crowded places because of fears that other people are looking at and negatively evaluating him or her? (G, C)	☐	☐
14. Very anxious around children he or she doesn't know well (or refuses to be around them)? (G)	☐	☐
15. Preoccupied with the possibility of vomiting in front of other people? (C)	☐	☐

Social anxiety disorder also affects kids' lives differently. Some children—particularly those with the generalized form of the disorder—can be severely hampered in many areas of their functioning. Kids who have multiple circumscribed social phobias may also often find that their lives are disrupted in a similarly serious way.

With these variations in mind, let's now look at four children who all have social anxiety disorder but are manifesting it in diverse ways.

Zoe

Zoe is mortified. Her teacher is going to require all of the students to give an oral report during the school year. In the past Zoe has been able to avoid situations like this by having her mom talk to the teacher and make other arrangements. But unlike her past teachers, her fifth-grade teacher won't accept a written assignment in place of a presentation.

Giving an oral report isn't the only situation Zoe is terrified of. She can't do other things that involve performing in front of people. Take last summer, when she had a part in the camp play. She was fine at all the rehearsals, but on opening night she froze up and couldn't go through with it. And at her piano recital she panicked and ran off the stage.

It's clear that Zoe has social anxiety disorder. Several performance situations—speaking in front of the class, acting in front of an audience, playing at a recital—make her extremely anxious. Like all kids who have social phobias, she's afraid she'll do something or say something "wrong" and end up being embarrassed. And because her public speaking anxiety is so severe, Zoe is already planning on "faking sick" and not going to school the day she's supposed to give her presentation.

In fact school refusal is not uncommon among kids who have social phobia. Fortunately in Zoe's case the event at school that makes her not want to go is going to happen only once this year. But as she goes on with her education and the requirements for public speaking increase, she's really going to have a problem unless she gets some help for her anxiety disorder.

Since Zoe has the circumscribed type of social phobia and her fears focus on performance situations, her social life is not that affected, unlike kids who have

> **School refusal is not uncommon among children who have social anxiety disorder.**

the generalized form of the disorder. She has many friends and is involved in a lot of social activities after school and on weekends.

Drew

Drew started kindergarten three months ago. At the beginning of the year his teacher wasn't that concerned about his behavior—lots of kids are shy and quiet when they first start school. But at this point Drew really should have adapted, and the fact that he hasn't suggests something is wrong.

Drew doesn't speak to anyone at school—not his teacher, his classmates, or any of the staff in the building. When spoken to, he usually tucks his head down to his chest and turns away. If he has to respond to a question, he nods, shakes his head, or uses hand signals to communicate.

Drew isn't just uncomfortable at school. He's anxious in other situations where he's around people he doesn't know well. When he was out with his mom and she ran into one of her friends, he tried to hide behind her. He refuses to go with his family to the neighborhood's block parties. And he's the only child on his street not using the new playground at the community center.

There's no doubt that Drew has the generalized form of social anxiety disorder. He's anxious in most social situations, with both kids and adults. When he can, he avoids situations where he'll be around people, particularly if he doesn't know them very well. But when he has to be in one of these situations—like at school—he's extremely uncomfortable.

Drew also has another problem that sometimes occurs in kids who have generalized social phobia. He won't talk—at all—at school. This condition, called *selective mutism* (see the sidebar on the next page), usually comes on before the age of five but often doesn't get identified until kids begin going to school.

As for many young children who have generalized social anxiety disorder, Drew's entire social life revolves around his family. At five this isn't such a big deal, but as he gets older and falls further behind in his social development, it will be. That's why now is the right time to take steps to help him overcome his problem.

Margo

Nine-year-old Margo is absolutely petrified that she's going to throw up in front of other people. The problem began back in first grade when she got sick all over herself right in the classroom. Even though it hasn't happened since then, one time was more than enough. She can't shake the idea that it will happen again.

Because she's so worried about the possibility of vomiting, Margo won't eat breakfast before going to school—she figures having an empty stomach will reduce the chance of throwing up. For a long time she wasn't eating anything at lunch either, but after much coaxing from her mom she now will have a very small amount of one of

Why Johnny Won't Speak

Some children refuse to speak in school, even to their classmates. This relatively rare disorder, known as *selective mutism*, is not caused by a speech or language problem. These kids have the ability to speak normally and do, like when they're home with their families.

Many children who have selective mutism develop a kind of "sign language" to communicate, using gestures and hand signals, and nodding or shaking their heads to express themselves. Others use their voices in a very limited way, responding to questions with guttural sounds or whispering monosyllabic—"yes," "no"—answers.

Although many children with this disorder also have social anxiety disorder—particularly the generalized type—the treatment for the two problems is not the same. So if you suspect your child has selective mutism, please make sure you seek the assistance of a child psychiatrist or psychologist who has experience in working with kids like this, who will be aware of and able to administer one of the many highly effective treatments that are available for this condition.

her "safe foods," foods she thinks are unlikely to cause a stomach problem.

Margo won't eat in restaurants, when she's at birthday parties, or in other situations where she's with people other than close family. She even refused to eat dinner when she went to her grandma and grandpa's last Christmas because out-of-town relatives she didn't know well were there.

Margo has a circumscribed social phobia about vomiting. She's afraid that what happened in the first grade is going to happen again, so she tries to limit her food intake, thinking this will decrease the likelihood that it will occur. As she's said to her mom, "If I don't eat, I can't throw up."

Margo's fear of vomiting is a social phobia because her primary concern is about how *embarrassed* she would be if she threw up in front of other people. Other kids have fears of vomiting that aren't social phobias—the fear is of the discomfort of the physical act itself, not public embarrassment (we'll discuss this further when we get to specific phobias in Chapter 8).

Margo's refusal to eat in public is connected to her phobia of vomiting; it's not another social phobia. There are children who do have social phobias about eating in front of others, but these kids are afraid that something about the way they eat will "look funny." Unlike Margo, they're not worried about throwing up.

Even though Margo's phobia is circumscribed, it's having significant effects on her life. Her limited food intake is affecting her energy level and interfering with her ability to concentrate in class. It's also causing her to be quite underweight, which could have health consequences down the road.

Leo

Twelve-year-old Leo's most valued possession is his computer. With the exception of going to school, he spends almost all his time online. In chat rooms and interactive games he's met a lot of kids, and he considers them to be his friends.

But in the real world—the one outside cyberspace—Leo doesn't have any friends. Although he's able to communicate well with a keyboard and computer screen, when it comes to real-life face-to-face

*encounters he completely falls apart. He's very nervous and awk-
ward around kids his age, not knowing what to say or how to act.
He's even uncomfortable on the telephone, though no one sees him
then.*

*The kids at school consider Leo to be an "oddball" and tease him
unmercifully, making his situation even worse. He doesn't want to
go school anymore and pleads with his parents, "Please let me be
home schooled!" But so far they've refused.*

Being hampered with generalized social anxiety disorder, Leo has
found a nonthreatening way to have some level of social interaction
(albeit very limited) via his computer. He's completely comfortable
and quite adept communicating in this way. Unfortunately, talking to
or being around other people is an entirely different story.

It's not unusual for kids with generalized social anxiety disorder
to have problems with social skills, and the fact that the kids at
school consider Leo an "oddball" raises the possibility that this may
be true for him (later on we'll discuss this subject in much more
depth). Children with generalized social anxiety disorder who do
not have social skills problems usually are described by other kids
as "shy"—not odd—and while they may be overlooked by their
peers (because they're so quiet), they're usually not teased or ostracized.

**Some children with
generalized social
phobia have social
skills problems.**

Leo's parents are wise not to allow him to
be home schooled. Further limiting his exposure to kids his age will most likely make his
social anxiety disorder worse. On the other
hand, continuing to be ridiculed by the students at his school is not
helping matters either. Perhaps the best solution will be to find an
alternative school for Leo offering an environment that will be more
accepting of him. Then he can take the steps he needs to overcome
his problem.

Situations That Can Cause Social Anxiety Disorder

At the very beginning of this chapter I spoke about how shyness in
young children can progress, intensify, and lead to social anxiety

Facts about Social Anxiety Disorder

The disorder is *equally common* in boys and girls.

Although children of any age can develop social anxiety disorder, the most typical time is during the *preteen years*, just following the onset of puberty.

After separation anxiety disorder, social phobia is the most common anxiety disorder diagnosis among children who *refuse to go to school.*

Public speaking is the most common circumscribed social phobia in both children *and* adults.

Many children with social anxiety disorder have *generalized anxiety disorder* too.

Children with social anxiety disorder are at risk for developing *depression*, particularly during adolescence.

---

disorder. However, although a large number of children with this anxiety disorder have a history of shyness, not all do. In fact some kids are perfectly fine socially until "something happens."

Mackenzie, a fifth grader, has always loved being the center of attention. Described by her parents as a "natural-born actress," she takes on almost any opportunity to perform. But when a case of food poisoning caused her to be sick

> **Kids who don't have a history of shyness can develop social anxiety disorder through learning experiences.**

during her school play, her performance days were over. Now she's terrified of doing most anything that places her center stage.

Ivan's parents weren't happy with the quality of education at the public schools in their area. Unable to afford private school, they decided to home school him instead. Although he did okay academically, Ivan felt isolated and lonely. When his folks finally put him back into public school, Ivan, who previously had no social problems, now was socially anxious.

Abigail has always been chubby but was never self-conscious about her weight. That was until fourth grade, when a group of girls began teasing her—calling her "the human blimp," "tubby," and other insulting names. Now Abigail, who has always loved school, doesn't want to go. She no longer wants to be around any other girls, not just the ones at her school, because she's worried they'll criticize her too.

Nine-year-old Simone has always been outgoing and had a lot of friends. But when her family moved to another town and she had to go to a new school (in the middle of the school year!), she became a completely different child—quiet, withdrawn, self-conscious, and uncomfortable with other kids.

All of these children—Mackenzie, Ivan, Abigail, and Simone—developed social anxiety disorder acutely, or suddenly, as a result of a specific situation. None of them previously were shy or overly self-conscious. Unlike other kids who seem almost biologically slated to develop this disorder (because of a slow, progressive pattern of shyness that's apparent from very early on), these children "learned" to be socially anxious because of unfortunate circumstances that made them that way.

Of course some children seem to have a combination of biological and experiential factors that come together and bring on the disorder. Remember Ashton? She always was shy but didn't have social anxiety disorder until her family moved and she started attending a new school. Would she have just remained shy and not developed an anxiety disorder if she had stayed in her old familiar surroundings? That's one of the topics we'll address next as we talk about ways to help prevent shy kids from developing social anxiety disorder.

Stopping Social Anxiety Disorder before It Starts: What to Do If You Have a Shy Child

Research has shown that shy children are at increased risk for acquiring social anxiety disorder. If your son or daughter has a shyness problem but doesn't have social anxiety disorder, you can do a number of things to decrease the likelihood that this will happen to your child. Although no one can give you a 100 percent guarantee that your child's shyness won't progress to an anxiety disorder, taking the steps outlined below will definitely help improve his or her chances.

1. Avoid abruptly changing your child's social environment.

There are certain situations that you need to be on the lookout for because they can exacerbate your child's problem. Moving to a new neighborhood and/or changing schools are two of them. Although both of these situations can be stressful for any child, they tend to be particularly traumatic for shy children.

If at all possible, don't move or change your child's school during the course of the school year.

If you have a shy child and you are considering making one of these changes, I advise you to seriously consider the potential consequences for your child when coming to your decision. If a move or school change is unavoidable, try to do it before the new school year begins (even if your child is not shy, it's a good idea to make the change at this time rather than during the course of the school year). Being the new kid in the class is tough enough without the additional attention and stress that come with first entering a classroom after school has been under way for a while.

2. Be vigilant about bullying or teasing at school.

If you have a shy child who all of a sudden doesn't want to go to school (or even if your child is not shy but abruptly becomes reluctant to go), find out if he or she is being teased by any of the kids in the class. You can talk to your child about this ("Is anybody being mean to you at school?") and also the teacher. If this is going on, make sure you help your child take care of the problem *right away*. This can mean working with your child on how to confront the bullies, asking the school to intervene, or speaking directly to the parents of the kids who are bothering your child.

In almost all cases one of these measures (or some combination of them) will work. But in the very unlikely event that none of them does, consider changing schools. Even though, as I said before, entering a new school is difficult for shy children, the discomfort it causes usually does eventually go away as kids get used to the new people and surroundings. By contrast, the discomfort that comes from relentless teasing does not go away. To the contrary, it's the kind of behavior that often leaves scars—of the social anxiety kind—that last a lifetime.

3. Don't allow your child to avoid performance situations.

Shy children often are reluctant to participate in activities that have them center stage—where other people's attention is focused on them. If your child is like this, it's important to encourage him or her to take on these challenges even though they may create feelings of anxiety. Communicate to your child that it's normal to have anxiety before an event like this ("anticipatory anxiety") and also for the first few minutes of the performance, but that the nervousness then almost always goes away.

If your shy child unfortunately has an unsuccessful experience performing at something—for example, messes up at the piano recital or gets tongue-tied giving a presentation at school—there are a couple of things you can do to help prevent it from possibly turning into a phobia. First try to reframe your child's experience using positive terms. For instance, if anxiety interfered with your child's ability to perform, try pointing out how great it is that he or she went ahead with the event despite the feelings or that the important thing is that your child tried—not the outcome. Reinforce how very proud you are of your child for doing something you know was difficult.

Another very important tack to take is to encourage your child to "get right back on the horse again." When kids have performance experiences they perceive as failures—especially when they are shy kids—their tendency is to want to avoid similar situations in the future. Please don't let your child do this! Avoidance is the surest way to create a phobia. Instead of allowing your child to avoid performance situations, encourage your child to participate in *even more* events like this and *as soon as possible*. Although it may not be possible to do the exact same thing—as in the case of a piano recital that occurs only once a year—your child will benefit almost as much from taking part in other performance-type experiences.

4. Make sure your child has ample social interactions with a variety of kids his or her own age.

I can't emphasize enough how important it is to stay on top of your child's social activities. Shy kids need to have ample opportunities to interact with other kids, and not just during the day at school. Make sure your child is scheduled for play dates after school or on the weekends and participates in other activities that include children who are the same age (interacting with younger or older kids does not have the same value as interacting with same-age peers).

Because shy kids often are reluctant to spend time with other kids—both individually and in groups—the way parents go about suggesting these activities can greatly influence the results. For example, it's often more effective to ask shy children which one of two activities they'd rather participate in than to ask them if they want to do something. (When you ask a child to choose, "no" is not a logical response. But when you ask a child whether he or she wants to do something, you're asking for a "yes" or "no" answer. Unfortunately in the case of a shy child the response almost always will be a "no.")

When Calvin's mom asked him whether he wanted her to schedule him a play date with Alex, he responded with a "no." But the next week when she tried again, this time following my suggestion ("Calvin, would you rather I schedule you a play date with Alex or with Eric?"), she was successful (he picked Alex). Marielle's mom had a similar experience with her child. Five-year-old Marielle, who previously had refused all of her mother's suggestions for after-school group activities, picked ballet when given the choice between it and soccer.

5. Increase your child's self-confidence in other areas.

Most shy children have a self-confidence problem. While following the suggestions I've just given you for social and performance situations will go a long way in helping your child, I've found it's also important with kids like this to work on developing feelings of competence in *nonsocial* areas. That's because the increased perception of self-worth gained from these activities often spills over into the social arena, making children more confident and able to take risks in their interactions with other kids. Fostering confidence in nonsocial areas also can carry over and increase self-confidence in performance situations too.

Fostering competence in <u>nonsocial</u> areas also can increase confidence in social and performance situations.

Is there some activity that your child has a particular proclivity for? Do you suspect there are natural abilities in a certain area? Is your child artistic, musical, athletic, a wiz at computers? Whatever the talent or interest, try to do everything you can to foster it.

Overcoming Social Anxiety Disorder

Despite taking the steps outlined above and making your best efforts, you may find that your shy child goes on to develop social anxiety disorder. Or you may have a child who was never shy but unfortunately acquired social phobia through certain learning experiences, perhaps one of the ones I talked about earlier.

Regardless of how your child got this way, there are many things you and your family can do to help your son or daughter overcome this problem. The psychological techniques I've included here are the same ones cognitive-behavioral therapists use when working with kids like this—techniques that research has shown are very effective at alleviating this problem.

While all the cognitive-behavioral methods can be taught by parents to their children, there are some instances where it may be best to get additional help and guidance from a professional in the field. For instance, if your socially anxious child is refusing to go to school and nothing you do is working to turn things around, it's time to seek outside help. Or if your child is showing signs of depression (see Chapter 2, pages 49–51) in addition to social anxiety disorder (not uncommon in kids with this anxiety disorder), it's very important that you have your child seen by a doctor as soon as possible. As you know, there are certain serious risks that can be associated with depression. Also, it will not be possible for you to work successfully on your child's social anxiety until the mood problem improves.

For many kids with social phobias the cognitive-behavioral techniques are all that's needed to get them past the problem. However, should you find that your child is not responding to them, or not responding as well as you'd like, you may want to consider having a child psychiatrist do an evaluation to determine whether your son or daughter is a good candidate for medication. There now are several psychiatric drugs that have been proven to be very helpful for social anxiety disorder, especially when combined with psychological techniques like the ones included here. (Research has shown that the medications are much more effective when used in conjunction with cognitive-behavioral treatment, so please make sure that you and your child use the psychological techniques, even if your child should require medication.)

In fact, I've seen kids who initially didn't get very far with the cognitive-behavioral methods but then responded beautifully to them after getting on the right medication. That's because the medication lowered their anxiety just enough so that they could learn and benefit from the psychological, self-help procedures.

1. Have your child gradually face—and conquer—his or her fears.

As you might expect, the key ingredient to having kids get rid of their anxiety in social and performance situations is to have them face the situations they fear. However, with that being said, *how* children confront their fears—the particular method that's used—plays a tremendous role in determining whether they'll be successful.

The method that's been shown to be most effective is called

graduated exposure. I talked about using graduated exposure for separation anxiety in Chapter 4 and for obsessive–compulsive disorder in Chapter 6. With this approach children are gradually exposed to situations that cause increasing levels of anxiety, beginning with ones that trigger only a little bit of discomfort and then proceeding, in a stepwise manner, to those that cause more and more discomfort.

The Social Anxiety Questionnaire you filled out earlier told you which phobia(s) your child has. The fear list and fear scale in Chapter 4 (see pages 107 and 108; extra copies of the fear list form are at the back of the book) will help you and your child come up with the steps that will be used for the graduated exposure for each phobia. If your child has just one social phobia, the two of you will need to create only one fear list. But if the Social Anxiety Questionnaire revealed that your child has more than one social phobia (either multiple circumscribed social phobias or generalized social phobia plus phobias of performance situations), you'll need to create separate lists, one for each phobia. (For kids who have multiple fear lists, please make sure you work on conquering one phobia—using *only one* list—at a time. Once that fear has been tackled, you and your child can move on to the next one.)

Remember Margo, the nine-year-old who was frightened she was going to throw up in front of other people? All of the items on Margo's fear list involve eating. Eating—when she's around, or anticipating being around, other people—makes Margo anxious because she believes it increases the likelihood that she'll throw up. Here's the fear list she and her mom created:

Margo's Fear List

Item 1 _Eating a small bag of pretzels for lunch at school_

Item 2 _Drinking juice before going to school_

Item 3 _Eating a piece of toast before going to school_

Item 4 _Eating cereal and milk or eggs and toast before going to school_

Item 5   _Eating a sandwich for lunch at school_

Item 6   _Eating cake at a friend's birthday party where you know all the kids_

Item 7   _Eating dinner at a restaurant with just your family_

Item 8   _Eating cake at a birthday party where you don't know all the kids_

Item 9   _Eating dinner at a restaurant with the soccer team after practice_

Item 10   _Eating dinner at a restaurant with your parents, their friends, and their friends' children (whom you don't know well)_

Looking at Margo's fear list, you can see that there are several different factors that seem to affect her level of anxiety: what type of foods and how much of them she eats, how "public" the setting is, and her familiarity with the people around her. Her worst situation, item #10—the one that makes her most anxious—is eating dinner (a lot of food) in a restaurant (a very public place) with kids she doesn't know well (unfamiliar).

Sienna is a third grader who has generalized social phobia. Her fear list is very different from Margo's. It focuses on situations that require social interaction. Let's take a look at her list, the one she and her mom worked on together:

Sienna's Fear List

Item 1   _Saying "hi" to a classmate_

Item 2   _Having a brief (less-than-five-minute) conversation with a classmate_

Item 3   _Raising your hand and answering one of your teacher's questions_

Item 4 _Raising your hand and asking your teacher a question_

Item 5 _Playing with at least one classmate at recess_

Item 6 _Having a child over for a play date_

Item 7 _Going to another child's home for a play date_

Item 8 _Having a sleepover at your home (just one child)_

Item 9 _Going to a birthday party where you know almost all of the kids_

Item 10 _Going to a birthday party where you know hardly any of the kids_

Your child's fear list will be different from Margo's and Sienna's, but the procedure for conducting the gradual exposure will be the same. Beginning with item 1 (the easiest one), arrange for your child to be in this situation as often as possible until it no longer causes anxiety. Keep in mind that it's repetition that makes anxiety go down, but this won't happen if the exposure practices are spaced too far apart. Daily practices are best (until the anxiety from the situation subsides), but if this isn't possible because of the nature of the item or other feasibility issues, try for at least once or twice a week. For example, the first five items on Sienna's fear list—all of which involve interacting with children at school—potentially could be practiced on five consequent (school) days in a single week. Items 6, 7, and 8, which involve play dates and sleepovers, probably could be done anywhere from one to three times in a week, while items 9 and 10—birthday parties—are something that can't be arranged in the same way the other situations can. To work on these situations Sienna and her mom will have to wait for opportunities to arise.

Once item 1 is no longer a problem, your child can move on to item 2. Again arrange for the exposure to the situation described in the item to occur as frequently as possible until it no longer causes anxiety. After this, have your child tackle each of the subsequent items on the list—one by one—until the final one, item 10, is accomplished.

In working with your child's fear list, please make sure you *do not have your child move on to a more difficult situation (the next item) until the current item no longer triggers any discomfort.* If you make this mistake, it's possible for your child to get worse rather than better! It's definitely better to repeat a step more times than is necessary than to take a chance on moving through the fear list too quickly.

It probably will take your child more exposure practices to become comfortable with the higher—more anxiety-provoking—items on the list. That's okay! It doesn't matter how long it takes for your child to get through the fear list, it only matters that he or she eventually does.

> **When doing gradual exposure, don't move on to a more difficult situation until the one your child currently is working on no longer causes anxiety.**

If your child gets stalled at one item on the fear list because he or she can't tolerate the exposure—the anxiety causes too much discomfort for the child to face the situation at all or to stick with it—keep reading. Your child can learn coping techniques like relaxation and positive self-talk (see strategies 2 and 4 below).

2. Teach your child relaxation techniques.

Although relaxation methods play a part in the treatment of many of the childhood anxiety disorders, they are particularly important for kids who have social anxiety disorder. Children with this disorder tend to spiral into a "negative feedback loop" after they experience physiological signs of anxiety in social or performance situations. They overreact to their physical symptoms because they are so concerned about others seeing them. This then causes them to get more anxious, which in turn makes their physical symptoms even worse.

This is what happens to Gavin when he has to speak in front of the class. He sees his hands trembling and worries that the other kids are seeing it too, which then increases his anxiety and causes the shaking to get worse.

Nine-year-old Elisa has a social phobia of blushing. When she feels some warmth on her cheeks, she's concerned they're turning red and someone will notice it. This causes her to become more nervous, which then increases the flush on her face.

Relaxation techniques reduce autonomic nervous system arousal and can help prevent or diminish physical symptoms of anxiety, like the ones Gavin and Elisa experience. But even if your child does not have anxiety symptoms that are clearly visible, relaxation techniques can get rid of overall feelings of tension and nervousness that can stand in the way of your child's confronting the situations he or she fears.

There are two different relaxation methods that I find work well with children. The first, *deep breathing*, involves learning to breathe slowly and deeply from the diaphragm. The second, *deep muscle relaxation*, involves tightening and then relaxing different muscles in the body.

Each of these relaxation methods has been discussed in depth elsewhere in this book—deep breathing in Chapter 4 (see pages 111–112) and deep muscle relaxation in Chapter 5 (see pages 138–140)—so I won't repeat what I've already said again here. However, please don't underestimate the importance of having your child learn these relaxation skills just because they're described in chapters devoted to other childhood anxiety disorders. As I said at the start of this section, although relaxation techniques are helpful to kids with many different types of anxiety problems, they're *especially* useful to children who have social anxiety disorder.

The relaxation skills can be used in conjunction with the graduated exposure exercises we talked about in the previous section. They can be used before the exposure to reduce anticipatory anxiety and also during exposure sessions to help keep anxiety at bay.

Ten-year-old Violet gets very nervous when she has to be in crowded places like the auditorium at school. She feels like the other kids are looking at her and they'll see that something is "wrong" with her. So before lining up to go into the auditorium Violet begins doing her deep breathing to keep her anxiety down. And once seated in the room she again turns to her breathing exercises to help keep her relaxed. For Violet, just like for many other kids who have social anxiety disorder, relaxation skills have played an important role in getting her through a difficult situation.

3. Improve your child's social skills.

Remember Leo, the child with generalized social phobia who was teased for being an "oddball"? There's no question that Leo is anxious interacting with other kids. But is it his anxiety that's causing the social problems or is it his lack of "social finesse" that's causing him to be anxious?

Children with the generalized form of social anxiety disorder fall into two groups. Some kids who have the disorder have perfectly fine social skills—they know how to interact appropriately with other people, but their anxiety impedes them from using their skills. In social situations they "freeze up" or "blank out," which can make them look socially inept, but if you see them with family or others they're comfortable with it's apparent they don't have a problem in this area.

Other kids with generalized social phobia, though, do have social skills problems. They lack the social knowledge and abilities needed to successfully interact and connect with people. They appear socially inept and awkward because *they are* this way, and being this way (which they are painfully aware of) causes them to feel anxious.

Like Leo, boys and girls who have social skills deficits appear—to a greater or lesser degree—as somewhat "off" or "odd." They seem oblivious to the social cues and subtle nuances of behavior that guide other children's social responses. They lack the "social rhythm" in their verbal and nonverbal behavior that flows almost effortlessly for most children. They usually are ostracized, and if they have any friends they too often have social skills problems.

If your child has the generalized form of social phobia (which you should know from your earlier answers to the Social Anxiety Questionnaire on page 181), it's important for you to know if there is a social skills problem. If there is, you'll need to address it by working on the development of these skills if you want your child's social anxiety to get better.

Completing the questionnaire on the next page will help you determine whether your child has a social skills problem. When completing the questionnaire, please be sure to answer each of the questions *twice*—the first time for how your child behaves with same-age children he or she knows well, the second time for how your child behaves with same-age children he or she *doesn't* know well.

A "yes" response to any of the questions indicates it's probably a problem area for your child. However, to really see if your child's behavior is due to a skills deficit (rather than anxiety hampering the expression of skills that your child really does possess), you will need to look over the general pattern of your answers to the questionnaire. Do the problems occur *regardless* of how well your child knows other children? In other words, when you answered with a "yes" to a question, did you do so for both situations—when with familiar and unfamiliar children? If this is the case, it's likely your child has some genuine weaknesses in social skills. On the other hand, problems that occur only when your child is with children he or she doesn't know well are probably due to anxiety rather than a skills deficiency (if your child is truly lacking a social skill, it will be absent regardless of his or her level of familiarity with others).

> **When socially anxious children have trouble communicating with <u>both</u> familiar and unfamiliar people, they probably have a social skills problem.**

The items in the questionnaire cover two general areas of social behavior that frequently are problematic for kids who have social anxiety disorder: nonverbal aspects of communication (questions 1 through 6) and speech content (questions 7 through 10). Take another look at your responses and see which (if either) of these areas is showing up as a problem. This will tell you what types of skills your child needs help with.

Lucas's mom completed the questionnaire and discovered that her eight-year-old son has trouble with some of the nonverbal aspects of communication. He has poor eye contact and speaks very softly. Rebecca, age ten, doesn't have these problems, but she has

Does Your Child Have a Social Skills Problem?

	Yes	No

1. Does your child have trouble looking directly at others either when speaking to them or when being spoken to?
   - With children he or she knows well? ☐ ☐
   - With children he or she doesn't know well? ☐ ☐

2. Is your child's voice often inappropriately loud or soft—the volume doesn't match the setting or situation—or does he or she speak in a monotone?
   - With children he or she knows well? ☐ ☐
   - With children he or she doesn't know well? ☐ ☐

3. Does it take your child too long to respond to others when they speak to him or her?
   - With children he or she knows well? ☐ ☐
   - With children he or she doesn't know well? ☐ ☐

4. Does your child's speech tend to have a lot of hesitancies in it—like pausing frequently or saying "ah" or "um" often?
   - With children he or she knows well? ☐ ☐
   - With children he or she doesn't know well? ☐ ☐

5. Does your child have poor posture or "body language" when speaking to other kids?
   - With children he or she knows well? ☐ ☐
   - With children he or she doesn't know well? ☐ ☐

6. Do your child's facial expressions often "not match" what's being said to him or her—like having a blank look when someone is saying something funny or smiling in response to a sad story?
   - With children he or she knows well? ☐ ☐
   - With children he or she doesn't know well? ☐ ☐

7. Does your child have difficulty expressing his or her feelings—either positive or negative?
   - With children he or she knows well? ☐ ☐
   - With children he or she doesn't know well? ☐ ☐

8. Does your child say things that don't follow from what others have just said?
   - With children he or she knows well? ☐ ☐
   - With children he or she doesn't know well? ☐ ☐

9. Does your child seem not to know what to talk about with other kids—have trouble making "small talk"?
   - With children he or she knows well? ☐ ☐
   - With children he or she doesn't know well? ☐ ☐

10. Do your child's verbal responses tend to be short?
    - With children he or she knows well? ☐ ☐
    - With children he or she doesn't know well? ☐ ☐

another type of social skills weakness. She doesn't know what to say to other kids.

Like the parents of these children, now that you know where your child's social weaknesses lie you can begin working to improve these skills. Kids can learn social skills by imitating a model (in this case you, the parent), through role playing (again, with you), and/or through gentle prompting paired with praise. Once a skill has been practiced sufficiently in a "safe" environment your child will need to try it out in the real world—that is, with other children.

Lucas's mother starting working on her son's problems by first concentrating on eye contact. When conversing with him she would remind him to look directly at her, and, then, after doing so, she immediately followed up with verbal praise ("Good!"). After a couple of weeks at this she found she rarely had to prompt Lucas at all—good eye contact was now becoming a habit, something Lucas was doing automatically.

The next thing that needed to be addressed was the volume of Lucas's speech. To get him to talk louder, his mom used both imitation and role-playing techniques. She started by having Lucas repeat short sentences she would say until his voice reached the appropriate degree of loudness. Here's a sample of what they did:

Mom: I like ice cream (*spoken in a moderately loud voice*).

Lucas: I like ice cream (*spoken in a very soft voice*).

Mom: Okay, Lucas, a little louder this time—"I like ice cream."

Lucas: I like ice cream (*a little louder, but not loud enough*).

Mom: That was a little better, but it still needs to be louder. Repeat after me—"I like ice cream."

Lucas: I like ice cream (*now spoken at the correct volume*).

Mom: That was great. Now let's just keep doing it a few more times to make sure you really have the hang of it. "I like ice cream."

Lucas: I like ice cream (*again, correct volume*).

Mom: Good. Again, "I like ice cream."

Lucas: I like ice cream (*still correct volume*).

Mom   Great. One last time—"I like ice cream."

Lucas: I like ice cream *(volume remains good).*

After doing well with these exercises, the next step was to get Lucas to use the louder speaking voice during conversations. To do this he and his mom set aside ten minutes each day to practice. During the practice time he and his mom would have a conversation (usually on a subject selected by Lucas) and Lucas would try to use his louder voice. If he inadvertently slipped back into speaking with his soft voice, Lucas's mom would point this out so he could make the correction. Just like when they worked on eye contact, after a couple of weeks Lucas made tremendous progress—he was speaking louder almost all of the time, not just during the practice sessions.

As you'll recall, ten-year-old Rebecca has a different problem than Lucas. Her nonverbal social skills are fine, but she has trouble with the content of her speech, which makes having conversations with other kids very difficult. To help her daughter strengthen her conversational skills, Rebecca's mom worked with her to come up with a list of five topic areas that would be of interest to the other girls in her class (and potentially good sources of conversation). Here is Rebecca's list:

1. Homework
2. Tests
3. Weekend activities
4. TV shows
5. Computer/Internet

After coming up with the list Rebecca and her mom started practicing having conversations using these topics. Using the role-playing technique Rebecca's mom pretended she was one of the girls in Rebecca's class and Rebecca, of course, was herself.

For her first practice session Rebecca chose the topic "weekend activities." With her mom's encouragement she initiated and maintained a conversation on this subject with her "classmate" for five minutes. The same task was repeated until Rebecca's side of the conversation was very smooth.

For the next couple of weeks Rebecca and her mom continued to work on Rebecca's conversational skills daily, selecting topics from her list. The practice definitely paid off—as the days went by Rebecca became more and more proficient at making small talk.

After Lucas and Rebecca made progress working with their moms, it was time for them to try out their new skills with other kids. Although it took some time, I'm happy to say that both of these children were able to transfer what they learned in their practice sessions at home to the outside world.

Just like Lucas and Rebecca's moms, you can work with your child to enhance whatever social skills are lacking and then encourage and monitor your child's use of these skills with other kids. How do you monitor your child's social behavior with other children? To find out how things are going at school you can speak to your child's teacher or just ask your son or daughter about it. When your child is in social situations outside of school you sometimes will be in a position to observe how he or she is doing yourself. Other times when you're not there you may be able to get feedback from other parents and adults (gymnastics teachers, soccer coaches, etc.).

Although I understand that some of you may have reservations about drawing the attention of others to your children's problems, when kids have social skills weaknesses it's apparent to the adults around them, so you won't be sharing anything with them that they don't already know. Also, it's really important that you keep abreast of how your child's social interactions are going. You want to make sure that your son or daughter continues to strengthen social skills *now* so he or she doesn't run into an *even greater* problem when the social demands increase later on, during adolescence.

4. Teach your child how to use positive self-talk.

As we saw earlier, a major part of social anxiety disorder is the negative thoughts children have about how others perceive them. While all of the techniques I've just described can be very effective at helping children overcome social anxiety disorder, they *will not work* if kids continue to anticipate and evaluate their behavior in social and performance situations as inadequate.

Juliana, age ten, thinks she's going to say something stupid when she's around other kids. During soccer practice eight-year-old

Terrence is afraid he'll miss the ball and be embarrassed in front of his teammates. Catherine, a third grader, is really anxious eating lunch around the other kids. She thinks, "What if food spills out of my mouth and I look like an idiot?"

Thoughts like these generate anxiety and prevent kids from becoming more comfortable in the situations they fear. Also, because they create anxiety the fears expressed in the thoughts can actually become a "self-fulfilling prophecy," making the very outcome your child dreads a reality. This is what happened to Scott, a sixth grader with a phobia of public speaking.

Scott was worried about giving his oral report. He was afraid he'd be so nervous that he literally wouldn't be able to speak. In fact he worked himself up so much beforehand with thoughts like these that by the time he got up in front of the class he was in a full-blown panic. When he began to speak, just like he feared, he couldn't get the words out—it was as if they were stuck in his throat. Scott's worst nightmare had come true.

Changing the negative, catastrophic thinking of social anxious children to more positive "self-talk"—thoughts that *reduce* anxiety—goes a long way toward helping kids overcome their fears. But before kids can make the switch to more helpful thoughts they need to be aware of their problematic thoughts while they are occurring.

> **Replacing negative, catastrophic thoughts with positive thoughts helps reduce anxiety.**

This may sound like a relatively simple matter, and in some cases it is. Many kids are very aware of their fearful thoughts as they are going through their heads, and when asked they are readily able to articulate them. But if this isn't true for your child, there are several ways you can help.

If your child tells you about his or her disturbing thoughts or says them out loud in your presence, you can point this out to make the thoughts more salient. Another way to help kids become more aware of their negative thoughts is to have them close their eyes and imagine they are in a social or performance situation that causes anxiety—preferably one they've recently experienced—and then have them relay what they are thinking.

Deion, a second grader, becomes extremely anxious whenever his teacher calls on him to answer a question. Since this just happened yesterday, Deion's mom thought today would be an especially good time to use the imagery method to get at Deion's negative thoughts. Deion's mom asked him to close his eyes, re-create the situation in his mind, and then—while imagining being in the situation—say out loud any thoughts that enter his head. Sure enough, after picturing the scene for less than a minute Deion said, "I won't know the answer to the question, and the kids will laugh!"

A third method—one that doesn't rely on having a parent around—involves having your child pay attention to when he or she is feeling anxious in a social or performance situation and then "backtracking" to the thoughts. I usually have kids carry a very small spiral notebook so they can write down the thoughts as they recall them. After doing this for a while children begin to be more aware of the thoughts as they are occurring, and then they no longer need to "backtrack."

Once the negative, catastrophic thoughts have been identified, the next step is to come up with positive, helpful thoughts that can be used to replace or counter the negative ones. The thoughts can be relatively general, coping-type statements, such as "I can handle this," "It's going to be okay," or "Nothing bad will happen."

While general, positive thoughts like those I just mentioned work well for many children, some kids find it's better to use specific thoughts that challenge the content of their negative thoughts. Let's take a look at this approach in action.

Catherine, mentioned on the previous page, has a social phobia about eating in public. She thinks that food will fall out of her mouth and she'll be embarrassed in front of the other kids. Here are the positive thoughts she and her mom came up with to counteract her negative thoughts:

1. It wouldn't be the end of the world.
2. It happens to other kids.
3. If it does happen, the kids will forget about it in a day or two.

You'll notice that Catherine's statements "downplay" or minimize what she fears, emphasizing that even if "the worst" happens it won't be catastrophic. Another useful strategy for creating positive thoughts is to have them focus on the low probability that what is feared will occur (obviously this approach is good only if the concern expressed in the negative thought really does have a small chance of happening). Using this approach, Catherine could have come up with a positive thought like this: "It [*sloppy eating in front of others*] hasn't happened since I was a little kid!"

Just like developing any new habit, it took a while for Catherine to get used to coming back at her negative thoughts with her new positive ones. At first using the method seemed a bit awkward and "forced," but with practice she became more comfortable with it. Eventually the positive self-talk seemed to come almost automatically. And as the positive thoughts increased, her social anxiety decreased. Today Catherine no longer has a problem eating in front of other kids.

Unfortunately I can't tell you what specific thoughts your child should use—to a large extent this will depend on what fears are expressed in your child's negative thoughts. But even when children have the same exact fears, it's possible that different types of thoughts will be more or less effective for them (for instance, some kids respond better to thoughts that deemphasize the *magnitude* of what they fear, while others respond better to ones that minimize the *likelihood* of what they fear). You can find out what works best for your child through trial and error, but generally I find that kids have a pretty good sense right away about whether or not a thought will do the trick for them. So when you're working with your child to develop the new thoughts, listen to what he or she has to say. In this particular case it's your child who most likely knows best.

As with the relaxation techniques I talked about earlier, your child should use positive self-talk in conjunction with graduated exposure, both before and during exposure sessions. You should also encourage your son or daughter to use the technique any other time he or she is experiencing social or performance anxiety and negative thoughts rear their heads.

Catherine was able to get control of her thoughts—and reduce her social anxiety—by using positive self-talk. With practice your child will too.

As you know from reading this chapter, one of the keys to overcoming social anxiety disorder is for kids to face the social and performance situations they fear. Together with social skills training to enhance social effectiveness and confidence, and relaxation and thought techniques to reduce anxiety, your child now has everything that's needed to get past this problem.

8 "MOMMY, DADDY, I'M AFRAID!"
Specific Phobias

Ten-year-old Carrie is afraid to sleep alone. In fact she never has slept by herself in her own room. She's uneasy in the dark and scared by the noises the house makes at night. "It sounds like someone is breaking in," she says.

When she was really little, Carrie slept in her parents' bed. After she started school, her folks tried to get her to move into her own room, but Carrie became hysterical. To calm her down, and as an "intermediate step," her mother decided to sleep alongside her daughter in the other bed in Carrie's room. But what started out as a temporary solution has turned into a permanent arrangement— five years later Dad is still alone in the master bedroom while Mom and Carrie sleep in the little girl's room.

At ten Carrie is definitely too old to have this problem. Is there anything her parents can do to get her past it?

As we discussed in Chapter 1, all kids have fears. There are certain times in your child's development when it's normal to be frightened of different things—like being afraid of small animals at three, four, or even five and getting terrified by thunder and lightning at six or seven.

But when fears persist beyond their usual developmental period—as for Carrie—they're no longer considered normal. And even if fears appear at "the right time," they still can be abnormal if they're severe enough. That's why, if your child has a fear that's age-inappropriate or excessive, you should consider the possibility that it's a phobia and not just a fear.

Although the normal fears of childhood are, by definition, transitory, specific phobias are not. If not attended to, they usually persist into adolescence and adulthood, where they can become even harder to get rid of. This happens in part because phobias tend to "spread" or "generalize" over time, which means that the number of situations that produce anxiety for your child keeps increasing.

Unlike the normal fears of childhood, specific phobias can have serious—even potentially debilitating—effects on children's lives. They can hamper your child's academic performance or interfere with social activities and friendships. In some cases specific phobias affect kids' ability to attend school, resulting in days, weeks, months, or—in extreme cases—even years of absences.

If your child has a phobia, there's no question that the sooner you address it the better. By intervening early you'll limit the effects of the disorder on your child now and also prevent things from continuing and worsening down the road. Later in this chapter you'll read about specific, detailed methods for your family to use to get your child past his or her phobia. But first it's a good idea to understand the characteristics of specific phobias so you can be sure this is what your child really is experiencing.

Diagnosing Specific Phobias

The criteria for diagnosing specific phobias are listed in the sidebar on the next page. As you can see, the characteristics of this anxiety disorder are similar to those of social phobia (see Chapter 7), except that in specific phobias the focus of the fear is not on social or performance situations and, as a result, children are not concerned about being embarrassed or humiliated. (Although, as we'll discuss later, they frequently have other kinds of disturbing or catastrophic thoughts about the objects and situations they're afraid of.)

To be diagnosed as having a specific phobia, your child's fear must be excessive or unreasonable. Please keep in mind, though, as I mentioned at the start of this chapter, that developmentally ap-

> Specific phobias are a lot like social phobias, except the fear isn't about a social or performance situation.

Symptoms of Specific Phobia

To be diagnosed with this disorder, a child has to have these symptoms:

- Persistently fears some thing or circumstance (besides the performance or social situations of social phobia) to an extent that is disproportionate to the situation or makes no sense.

- Either avoids or tries to avoid the feared thing, place, or event or experiences severe anxiety or distress when exposed to it.

- Either has some part of his or her daily life—school performance, social activities or relationships, normal routine—disrupted or is extremely upset about having the phobia.

propriate "normative fears"—the ones I talked about in Chapter 1—are not diagnosable as phobias unless the fear, even though age-appropriate, is more severe than what would be expected of a child of that age. (If you're not sure whether your child's fear is age-appropriate, you might want to review the timeline for normative fears on page 5 to refresh your knowledge about what's expected and considered normal at different ages.)

For instance, seven-year-old Julia can't go to sleep unless a nightlight is on in her bedroom and the light in the hallway is left on too. This is normal for a child her age. On the other hand, Niles's and Claudia's fears of the dark are not normal. Although Niles is the "right" age to have this fear (he's six), he can't do things that other kids his age can do—like go to the movies or enter a darkened room and turn on a light switch—because his fear is too excessive. Like Carrie, introduced at the opening of this chapter, Claudia, age twelve, should no longer be so afraid of the dark. But despite her age, she has to take her nightlight with her when she sleeps over at a friend's house.

It's also important to keep in mind that, unlike adults with specific phobias, kids don't always recognize that their fears are greater than they should be or that they don't make sense—it's often parents or other adults who identify them in this way. For example, Daniella, a third grader, thinks it makes sense to be afraid of dogs

("They can bite me!"), but her mom knows her daughter's fear has gone too far. Even when she comes across a dog that's leashed, Daniella insists on crossing the street to the other side.

Children can have specific phobias of almost anything. The most common ones, though, are of dogs, cats, and other small animals, insects, the dark, vomiting, going to school (we'll talk about this particular phobia at length later on), heights, plane flights, elevators and other enclosed places, deep water (swimming), and hypodermic needles. Because the content of specific phobias varies greatly, they usually are classified into "subtypes," with fears that share a similar theme being grouped together into the same category. In the chart below I've listed the subtypes, as well as examples of fears that fit into each one. As you can see, there are four main categories: animals/insects, medical/illness/injury, natural environment, and situational, plus an additional one for other, miscellaneous fears that don't clearly fit into any of the four main groups.

Regardless of the type of phobia, children react to being confronted with their fears with intense anxiety or distress. Some kids have full-blown panic attacks, while others have more limited or specific anxiety symptoms, like upset stomachs (sometimes to the point of vomiting), heart palpitations, or tremulousness. Some children (usually younger ones) show their distress by throwing tantrums, crying, or clinging. It's not unusual for kids to try to "run away" or escape from the situation (like Daniella, who crosses to

Types of Phobias

Animals/insects:	Cats, dogs, lizards, snakes, bees, spiders
Natural environment:	High places, thunderstorms, the dark, deep water
Medical/illness/injury:	Going to the doctor or dentist, needles, seeing blood, having an illness or injury, vomiting
Situational:	Flying, crowded places, elevators, enclosed places, tunnels, bridges, riding in a car
Other:	Loud noises, costumed characters

the other side of the street when she sees a dog), although other kids do just the opposite—they "freeze" and become immobilized.

Given the chance, almost all children with phobias will avoid what they fear altogether. But if they can't—usually because their parents won't let them—they'll face the situation and have the types of reactions just described.

It's important to emphasize that to be considered a phobia your child's fear needs to have significant, negative effects on functioning (like interfering with your son or daughter's ability to follow his or her normal routine or impacting academic performance, social activities, or relationships), or else your child must be extremely distressed about having the fear (in other words, your child is very upset that he or she has the problem). This is the way that relatively inconsequential fears—those that don't warrant a psychiatric diagnosis—are differentiated from phobic disorders (those that do warrant a psychiatric diagnosis and intervention). Since most kids (and adults too, for that matter) have fears, it's really important to make this distinction accurately.

It's clear that seven-year-old Mallory's fear of cats is severe enough to be considered a phobia. It's significantly affecting her life. She won't play outside with the other kids because there are cats that roam her neighborhood, and she refuses to visit her best friend's home because they have two cats as pets.

Carlos and Mary Beth also have fears that should be classified as phobias. Carlos, a fourth grader, is excessively fearful of getting sick. He tries to get out of going to school because he's afraid he'll pick up illnesses from his classmates. Mary Beth, a first grader, is so scared of the loud noises at school—the announcements on the intercom system, the school bell, and the alarm used for fire drills—that she's having trouble paying attention and isn't keeping up with the other students.

You might be interested to know that about half of children who have specific phobias develop the disorder after being involved in a distressing or traumatic incident or event or following exposure to upsetting information about the object or situation they come to fear. For instance, Sandy, a fourth grader, became terrified of elevators after she and her dad were trapped in one for ten minutes. Following a car accident, Rosie, age seven, developed a phobia of riding in cars. After watching a documentary show on the West Nile virus, eleven-year-old Dale developed a phobia of mosquitoes (a major problem since he lives in the South, where he's exposed to them pretty much all year). Eight-year-old Vito became claustrophobic— fearful of small enclosed places—after his cousin locked him in a closet. Carolyn, a sixth grader, developed a phobia of needles and blood after learning about AIDS in health class.

The Many Faces of Specific Phobias

As you've just seen, specific phobias can take many forms. Some fears are about medical and health-related issues, others involve animals or insects, some focus on situations in the natural environment, while yet others involve special types of situations that often include a travel or claustrophobic component.

In addition to the different types of fears, the effects that phobias have on children's lives vary. Some kids are very distressed about having a phobia and experience a lot of anxiety but aren't significantly hampered in their ability to participate in their everyday activities. Other kids' phobias, though, more severely affect their functioning, even, in some cases, interfering with their ability to go to school.

With this in mind, let's look at four children who all have specific phobias but have very different ways of showing it.

Daniel

Daniel's mom has a big problem. Her nine-year-old son becomes hysterical at the prospect of going to the doctor or dentist. In fact, he gets so worked up that she doesn't tell him when he's going until an hour before the appointment. Although this has limited the amount of time during which he's upset, his reaction is still extreme—he throws a major tantrum and refuses to get in the car or else tries to run away. Ultimately, his mom has to physically force him to go, often enlisting the help of Daniel's father.

When asked why it's so upsetting to go, Daniel says, "I don't like the needles!" He's frightened of getting injections or having his blood drawn (even by a finger prick) at the doctor's, and can't tolerate the needle the dentist uses in his mouth to administer the anesthetic.

Many, if not most, children are afraid of the discomfort caused by needles. But in Daniel's case the fear is so severe that it meets the definition of a phobia. The fact that he has to be physically forced to go to the doctor or dentist—often requiring the involvement of both of his parents—attests to the intensity of this child's fear. And his overwhelming anxiety over even relatively minor situations involving needles—such as having his finger pricked—also supports the diagnosis. In addition to Daniel's problem with needles, he's fearful of other things he encounters in the doctor's and dentist's offices. For example, he's scared by the sound the drill makes when he has to get a cavity filled. He also is afraid of seeing blood (particularly his own, which may be part of the reason he reacts so strongly to having his finger pricked) and of vomiting.

It's not unusual for kids to have more than one phobia, and when they do the fears often fall into the same subtype.

It's not unusual for kids to have several specific phobias, and when they do—as for Daniel—the phobias often fall into the same subtype, in this particular case "medical/illness/injury." There are many things Daniel's parents can do to help their son get over his phobias, which we'll get to later in this chapter.

Ali

Eleven-year-old Ali is terrified of thunderstorms. The booming noise of the thunder and the loud crackle of the lightning send a chill up her spine. She's also frightened that the lightning will hit her or her house, so she refuses to go out—even to school—or to go to sleep during a storm.

Ali is so concerned about the possibility of thunderstorms that she checks the weather forecast many times each day. She's also on alert for hurricanes and tornadoes—even though they happen less frequently—because windstorms frighten her too.

If a thunderstorm unexpectedly occurs while she's at school, Ali goes into a panic. In fact she gets so anxious that she can't hear what the teacher is saying and isn't able to concentrate well enough to do her assignments.

It's clear that Ali's anxiety about storms is a phobia. At eleven she's definitely too old to be so scared of thunder and lightning. And even if her fear were age-appropriate (for instance, if she were five or six), it wouldn't be considered normal because of how it's impairing her functioning.

As we discussed earlier, almost any phobia can result in school avoidance. In Ali's case, her absenteeism occurs sporadically, because it depends on the weather, which varies from day to day. If her phobia centered on something that occurs every—or almost every—day, the amount of school missed would probably be much greater.

In addition to making her miss school, Ali's phobia at times affects her sleep and her ability to concentrate in school and keeps her from participating in her usual social activities. It also causes her a great deal of distress, and not only when a storm is occurring. Like many other kids with specific phobias, she's constantly "on alert" to the possibility of encountering what she fears, which is why she so frequently checks the weather forecast.

Like Daniel, Ali has more than one phobia (tornadoes and hurricanes, as well as thunderstorms), all of which fall into the same subtype ("natural environment"). Since tornadoes and hurricanes *are dangerous*, you might question whether they really should be considered *phobias*. Recall, though, that to be a phobia a fear must make no sense *or* be disproportionate (you might want to look again at the sidebar on page 210). Although Ali's fears of tornadoes and hurricanes are somewhat reasonable, they are excessive—she worries way too much about them, as her weather checking demonstrates.

> **To be a phobia a fear doesn't have to be unreasonable–it can just be excessive.**

Dayna

Dayna is claustrophobic. When her second-grade class had a field trip to an amusement park, she couldn't go on any of the rides that involved being in small, confined spaces—like the submarine ride and the "Tower of Terror" elevator ride. In fact, as far as elevators go, she always tries to get her family to take the stairs instead, because when she's in an elevator (unless it's the glass kind) she gets butterflies in her belly and feels really hot and sweaty. Because of her problem, Dayna also doesn't want to play some of the games her friends want to play, like "making a tent" and "hide and seek."

Dayna also is afraid of being in places that are very crowded. She's uncomfortable in the school auditorium and in church when these spaces are really packed. She doesn't like to go to sports events in crowded arenas or to the movies if the theater is full. She tells her mom that when she's in these situations, "I feel trapped and like I can't breathe."

There's no question that Dayna has several specific phobias—of elevators, other types of enclosed places, and crowded places—that all fall into the "situational" subtype. She tries to avoid the things she's afraid of, but if she can't—as when she has to go to the school auditorium or church—she endures them with tremendous anxiety and discomfort.

Claustrophobia, which is a fear of small, enclosed places (that often are without windows or light), can make kids (and adults who have this problem too) feel like they're trapped and can't get out of the situation they're in. It's also very common for children with this phobia—just like Dayna—to say that they feel they "can't breathe" or that they're not getting enough air. This sensation usually comes from hyperventilating—breathing too shallowly and rapidly. (Later on I'll be sharing with you a technique that you can teach your child if your son or daughter has this problem.)

It's not unusual for kids who have phobias of small, enclosed places also to have a phobia of crowded places. Even though crowded places aren't, by strict definition, considered to be "claustrophobic" situations, they can produce the same feelings of confinement—feeling trapped and unable to breathe—that are experienced in elevators or other small, windowless spaces. (As you know from the last chapter, a fear of crowded places isn't necessarily a specific phobia—it also can be indicative of a *social* phobia. It's a social phobia, and not a specific phobia, if the fear is of being observed by others and humiliated or embarrassed in some way. On the other hand, fears of being trapped and unable to get enough air—as for Dayna—are specific, not social, phobias.)

Evangeline

Evangeline is petrified of dogs. As far as she can remember, she's always been uncomfortable around them, but as she's gotten older (she's eight now), her fear has gotten much worse.

There are a lot of things Evangeline can't do, or is extremely uncomfortable doing, because of her fear. She won't have play dates at any of her friends' homes where there are dogs—to get together they have to come to her house. She won't go into pet stores because even if they don't sell puppies they sometimes allow customers to bring their own dogs inside. She says "no" when her friends want to take a bike ride in the neighborhood park because a lot of people walk their dogs there.

Evangeline's fear is so strong that she even has trouble with pictures of dogs, especially if they seem very lifelike. She turns away if she sees a dog in a movie or on TV and feels nervous if she sees a photograph of a dog or a picture of one in a book or in her Highlights *magazine.*

At eight, Evangeline is past the age where she should be frightened of dogs. In addition to not being age-appropriate, her fear is more severe than what would be expected of even a much younger child (say age four or five).

In addition to causing her a lot of distress, Evangeline's phobia is interfering with her relationships with other kids. She refuses to go over to the homes of her friends who have dogs (including, unfortunately, her three closest friends) and won't participate in certain group activities (like riding her bicycle in the park) with them. The strain this puts on her relationships is beginning to take its toll— her friends are calling her less frequently, preferring to get together with kids who don't impose the restrictions Evangeline does.

Unlike the other children we've just talked about, Evangeline has only one phobia. She's not afraid of any other types of animals or insects or any of the fears of the other phobia subtypes. Interestingly, Evangeline's mother has the exact same phobia that her daughter has—she's terrified of dogs too. As discussed in Chapter 3, sometimes kids learn to be anxious—and develop anxiety disorders like phobias—through observation. This might be what happened to Evangeline and could account for why she has only one phobia.

What Is "School Phobia"?

At some time or another you've probably heard the term *school phobia*. In reality, there really is no such thing as a phobia *of school*, per se. When kids are afraid to go to school, either they are scared of some aspect of the school environment or something that might happen at school or they have anxiety about leaving home or being away from their families (see Chapter 4 on separation anxiety disorder for more about this). The term *school phobia*, then, refers to an irrational, excessive fear of—and desire to avoid—attending school, which can stem from a number of sources.

As we discussed in the last chapter, many social and performance situations can cause children anxiety and lead them to try to avoid going to school. Specific phobias—especially certain, select ones that I'll be talking about shortly—also can result in school avoidance.

Brady, a fifth grader, is quite small for his age. Even though no one has threatened him, he's terrified that he's going to get beaten up by the other boys and wants to stay home from school. Eleven-year-old Diego also doesn't want to go to school. He's petrified of "picking up something"—a virus or more serious illness—there.

Facts about Specific Phobias

The disorder is *equally common* in boys and girls.

Most specific phobias begin in childhood, well *before* the onset of puberty.

Of all the childhood anxiety disorders, specific phobia is the *most common*.

It's not unusual for children to have *more than one* specific phobia. When they do, they often fall into the same "subtype."

Many children who have this disorder have other anxiety disorders too, particularly *social anxiety* or *separation anxiety disorder.*

Janice, age eleven, is very physically uncoordinated. She's scared she's going to get hurt in gym class and refuses to go to school on gym days.

You'll notice that the examples I've just given all involve the possibility of some type of harm happening to the children—getting sick or being physically attacked or injured. While this is the most common theme that results in school refusal in kids who have specific phobias, other types of specific phobias can cause kids to want to avoid school too. For example, seven-year-old Camilla, who has a phobia of dogs, doesn't want to go to school because of the stray dogs that are near the playground. Five-year-old Gunner also wants to stay home. He is scared of the time-out room—a very small, enclosed space that has no windows—that he gets put in if he misbehaves.

> **Although it's possible for almost any phobia to cause school refusal, fears of illness or injury are most likely to do so.**

Specific phobias like the ones I just talked about can make kids reluctant to go to school or cause them to miss occasional days of school. At the other end of the continuum, though, kids can be absent for weeks, months, or even—in extreme cases—years of school. If your child's phobia is beginning to cause a problem with going to school, you'll want to address it right away since significant absenteeism has many deleterious effects and not just on academic performance. Many of the intervention techniques I'll be discussing later can be very helpful for dealing with "school phobia," but if your child already is missing a lot of school, it's best to seek professional help for this problem.

Stopping Phobias before They Start: What to Do If You Have an Overly Fearful Child

Seven-year-old Jessica has many fears. Although she doesn't have any that are diagnosable as phobias, they still cause her and her family a lot of distress.

Some children, like Jessica, tend to be excessively fearful. They don't (at least not yet) have specific phobias—because their fears are

School Phobia or Truancy?

Adults can have a hard time comprehending the anxiety reactions of children. One of the best examples of this is when kids have phobias that affect their ability to attend school. What is there to be afraid of at school when there is nothing overtly dangerous there? In fact, because fears of going to school seem so far-fetched to some people, children with this problem can be labeled inaccurately and treated unfairly by the school system as truants or delinquents (kids like this don't have anxiety about going to school—they just prefer not to be there). When this happens, parents and their children can end up having to deal with the judicial system, rather than receiving the help they really need from the mental health system.

If your family encounters a problem like this, you're probably going to need the assistance of a mental health professional to educate school personnel (and members of the legal profession if things have gone that far) about phobias that cause school refusal and act as an advocate and liaison so your child can have a comfortable and successful return to school. Also, although the strategies I will discuss later can help with "school phobia," as for other specific phobias, when a child is missing a lot of school it's best to get outside, expert professional help to guide the treatment process.

either age-appropriate or just not severe enough to warrant a diagnosis—but they are more fearful (have higher fear levels) of more things (a larger number of objects and situations) than other kids their age.

Research has shown that children like this may be prone to developing specific phobias. However, if you have a son or daughter who is overly fearful, there are steps your family can take right now to decrease the likelihood that your fearful child will turn into a phobic child. Not only will you potentially be stopping a serious problem before it starts, you'll also be helping your child be more comfortable and function better today.

1. Encourage your child to approach—and not avoid—his or her fears.

It's a natural instinct for children (and adults too for that matter) to want to avoid or escape objects and situations that cause fear. While staying away from certain types of scary things is good because it has "survival value" (like running away from a wild animal or not jumping into deep water if you can't swim), other fears do not serve any useful purpose (although they might have at one time—see pages 8–9 in Chapter 1 for a discussion of the evolutionary value of fears).

Avoidance behavior strengthens fears, while approach behavior (if done correctly) diminishes them. That's why it's so important to encourage your child to face fears rather than running away from them.

How do you do this? Coaxing, in the form of gentle persuasion, and praise can be very effective. Some parents also find that using small rewards—material, tangible items or special activities or events—works well (once children conquer their fears, the rewards can be phased out). Another way to help encourage children to face their fears is to pair the scary situation with something positive that is likely to create good feelings. For instance, Bradley's mom has an "ice cream party" with her five-year-old son on nights when there's a thunderstorm. (It's also important to let children know that their fears will lessen the more often they confront them. As we'll talk about more in the next section, when it comes to overcoming fears the rule of thumb is "repetition, repetition, repetition." That's one of the reasons phobias that involve situations that are encountered infrequently often are harder to get rid of. Again in the next section, when we discuss conquering phobias, I'll share with you ways to get around this problem.)

2. Serve as a role model for your child by demonstrating nonfearful behavior and ways of thinking.

Parents can serve as role models for their kids by having their children first observe them successfully confronting the feared object or situation *and then* having kids try to duplicate the behavior. This approach worked well for Sharon, a third grader who was afraid of cats. Sharon's mom took her to a pet store and held a kitten for a couple of minutes, to show Sharon there was nothing to be afraid of. Then she asked Sharon to do the same. Although at first Sharon was a bit hesitant, with a little encouragement she held the kitten, and after a few minutes she was completely comfortable in the situation.

Five-year-old Aubrey's mom also successfully used this method to help her daughter with her fear of "monsters." Aubrey was having a problem going to sleep at night because she was afraid that monsters were hiding in her room. Although Aubrey's mother obviously couldn't literally confront the monsters (since they don't exist), she was able to approach the places that—in her child's mind—they might be lurking. By looking in the closet and under the bed a few nights in a row, Aubrey's mom was able to convince her daughter that her room was free of monsters, and, as a result, Aubrey quickly got over her fear.

> **By modeling approach behavior, parents can give their children the confidence to try it on their own.**

You can also help reduce your child's anxiety about what he or she fears and increase the child's confidence about approaching the situation by reframing it—giving your child another way to think about it—so it doesn't seem so frightening. For example, Billy's mom responded to her son's concerns with how much needles hurt by telling him "It lasts only a second!" Sheila's dad helped her with her fear of Scruffy (the friendly, but somewhat overactive, beagle living next door) by explaining his "doggy behaviors" in a positive (and more realistic) way:

Sheila: Dad, I'm scared that Scruffy is going to hurt me when he jumps up on me.

Dad: But that's Scruffy's way of telling you he likes you. That's the way that dogs say "hello."

Sheila: But what about when he goes to lick me? I'm afraid he's going to bite.

Dad: For doggies, licking is like kissing. It's another way that he's showing he likes you.

In Sheila's case her dad wasn't just reframing the situation; he was also giving her some information she didn't have before, information that could help lessen her fear. We'll be discussing the importance of providing educational material to children to help them overcome fears in more detail later on, when we talk about ways to get rid of phobias.

3. Use your child's action heroes as examples of courageous behavior.

Using action heroes—or other figures, real or fictitious, that your child admires—as examples of courageous behavior can be a very effective tool for combating fearfulness, particularly with younger kids. When your child confides in you that he or she is afraid to do something, you can respond with "How would _____ [*the real or imagined "hero"*] handle that?" or "What would _____ [*the real or imagined "hero"*] do in that situation?"

Roberto, age nine, is a big fan of Spider-Man. When he told his dad he was afraid of his friend's pet snake, his father asked, "How would Spider-Man deal with that?" Roberto thought about it for a few seconds and then replied, "He would tell the snake 'I'm bigger and stronger than you,' and he wouldn't be afraid." His dad then said, "Then I think you should try saying that same thing to yourself!" (Obviously, this is a good idea only if the snake is not poisonous or any kind of threat. I'm not suggesting children should be led to believe they have "super powers" or should confront dangerous situations!)

Six-year-old Joseph is enamored with Sponge Bob. When he became anxious about taking his first plane trip, his mom decided to use her son's favorite television character to try to increase his confidence in his ability to handle this new situation. Joseph's mother said, "I know that doing something you've never done before—like flying in a plane—can be scary. How would Sponge Bob handle a new situation like this?" To this question Joseph quickly replied, "Sponge Bob always has fun when he does something new!" "So why can't you too?" his mom asked. "Why can't you be just like Sponge Bob?" Using Sponge Bob as a "springboard" for Joseph to approach flying in a more positive way worked. He then began to actually look forward to the trip, planning fun things to do during the flight.

4. Work on increasing your child's self-esteem.

Being a fearful kid doesn't feel good. Overly fearful children often feel bad about themselves, suffering from low self-esteem. Since self-confidence can play a big part in motivating kids to demonstrate courageous behavior—facing their fears rather than avoiding them—working on increasing self-esteem can indirectly help kids conquer their fears.

> **Building self-confidence by acquiring new skills can help overly fearful children face their fears.**

Although many different kinds of activities can help kids feel good about themselves, becoming skilled at certain physical activities—like karate (or any of the other martial arts) or gymnastics—often is particularly effective at getting fearful children to develop a newfound sense of self-confidence. This probably is because of the sense of control that's obtained by mastering control of one's own body (that is, bodily movements).

Eight-year-old Rosa had a terrible fear of vomiting (in her case it was a specific phobia, not a social phobia, because she was fearful of the physical act of throwing up, not about the potential embarrassment she might suffer from doing it in front of others) and many other fears too. After reading this chapter, her mom decided to enroll her in a gymnastics class. After two months of classes, Rosa was like a different child. More confidence, less fearful—exactly what her mother had hoped to achieve.

Getting Rid of Specific Phobias

If you're reading this section, you either have a child who already has a specific phobia—so the guidelines I've given for prevention won't be appropriate for your family—or, despite your best efforts, your overly fearful child has gone on to develop a phobia. Regardless of which is the case, there are many things you and your child can do to turn the situation around. Specific phobias are not only the most common of the childhood anxiety disorders but are often the easiest to treat as well. Parents frequently are able to get their children's phobias under control on their own, without the assistance of a psychologist or other mental health professional and without psychiatric medication.

The psychological techniques included here are the very same ones that cognitive-behavioral therapists use to treat children with specific phobias. The overwhelming effectiveness of these methods has been documented by numerous research studies (literally in the thousands!), so you can be confident that you'll have exactly the right tools to take care of your child's problem.

Although all of the procedures I've included here can readily be used by parents with their children, in some instances it may be best to get outside help, either to assist you in your efforts or to serve in your place. As I said earlier in this chapter when discussing "school phobia," if your child's phobia is causing him or her to miss a lot of school, it really is in your child's best interest to obtain the assistance of a mental health professional who is a specialist in this area. And if you happen to have the same phobia as your child (not uncommon, as we discussed in Chapter 3), it may not be possible for you to work effectively with your son or daughter on the fear.

Finally, although self-help books go a long way in giving parents what they need to address their children's problems, some parents simply feel more secure using the techniques under the guidance of a trained professional. There's certainly nothing wrong with taking this approach, and, in fact, it might help to move things along faster. But if you do choose to do this, please make sure you and your child's doctor are "on the same page." Show the doctor this chapter so he or she will know exactly where you're coming from and what you are planning on doing to deal with your child's phobia.

1. Make sure your child has the facts.

Many times kids' phobias are based, at least in part, on misunderstandings. When this is the case, it's amazing the power that information can have on reducing their fears.

Jacob, a fifth grader, has a phobia of flying—well, really, the turbulence that can occur during flights. He thinks it means something is wrong with the plane and it's going to crash. When his dad had him speak with a pilot (a close friend of his father's), Jacob learned that turbulence is caused by air pockets in the sky, similar to waves in the ocean, and that the people who fly airplanes are very used to it (just like boat captains who are comfortable running their ships when there are waves). After his talk with the pilot, Jacob's fear of flying lessened dramatically.

Jody, age eight, is terrified of cats. She knows they're related to lions (which are "really big cats") and she's afraid that—just like lions—they'll attack her. Her mother stepped in and taught Jody about the difference between domesticated and wild animals. Armed with her new knowledge, Jody became much less frightened of cats.

Eleven-year-old Dominique is petrified of contracting AIDS. She steers clear of people who look like they are "homeless" or "bums" because she thinks she can pick up the disease from them. When Dominique learned in health class that AIDS is transmitted through the exchange of bodily fluids—and not through the air (as she had incorrectly believed)—and that AIDS has nothing to do with homelessness, her fear diminished.

Jacob, Jody, and Dominique's situations demonstrate the value of education in getting rid of irrational fears. All of these children had misinformation or misunderstandings about the things they were fearful of, and gaining correct information—"the facts"—worked wonders in lessening their fears.

2. Create a fear list and tackle the phobia one step at a time.

If you've read some of the other chapters in Part II, you know that this isn't the first time I've talked about using a fear list—and *graduated exposure*—to overcome anxiety disorders (Chapters 4, 6, and 7, on separation anxiety, obsessive–compulsive, and social anxiety disorders, respectively, all discussed the use of this method). But just in case you haven't read about it already, or to refresh your memory, I'll go into it again here now.

Graduated exposure, as the name implies, involves gradually exposing kids to the source of their phobia, beginning with situations that cause only a little bit of fear or anxiety and then slowly—step by step—moving on to increasingly difficult situations. The keys to using graduated exposure successfully are to:

1. Make sure you start with an exposure experience that triggers a *very minimal* level of anxiety;
2. Make sure subsequent "steps" (exposure assignments) are each *just a little bit harder* than the previous one; and
3. Have your child move on to a new step only once the exposure task he or she has been working on no longer causes any fear or anxiety (this is achieved by having your child repeat the same step as many times as is necessary for the fear to leave completely).

Using the form on the next page, write in the specific phobias your child has. Taking another look at the sidebar on page 211, which lists the fear types along with lots of examples, can help you be sure you don't miss any (although, if it's truly a phobia, it's unlikely you'll need to consult the list to recall your child's phobias—but you might want to look at it anyway, just to be sure).

If your child has more than one specific phobia (which, as I've said before, isn't at all unusual), you'll need two or more fear lists, one for each phobia. And if your child has multiple phobias, the two of you will need to decide which one to work on first.

There are generally two schools of thought on which way to go with this. The first school subscribes to the notion that the phobia that is the least severe—the one that causes the least distress and interference in your child's life—should be tackled first. The idea here is that the early, relatively easy success achieved with the least severe phobia will then help motivate your child to go on to tackle the more difficult ones. The second school of thought suggests that you start with the *most* severe phobia—the one that causes the greatest distress and interference in your child's life. The thinking here is that overcoming the worst phobia will yield the greatest rewards (positive change in your child's life), which will then help motivate your child to follow up and confront the remaining fears.

Personally, I don't think either one of these approaches is clearly better than the other. However, I do think that in almost all cases it's best to include your child in on the decision on which phobia to work on first. Because overcoming phobias—even using graduated exposure—is not all that pleasant, the more motivation you can

Your Child's Phobias

List all **animal and insect** phobias:

_____

_____

_____

List all phobias of the **natural environment**:

_____

_____

_____

List all **medical, illness, and injury** phobias:

_____

_____

_____

List all **situational** phobias:

_____

_____

_____

List any **other** phobias:

_____

_____

_____

elicit from your child, the better the outcome will be. However, if your son or daughter has a phobia that is seriously affecting very important aspects of his or her life—such as causing absences from school—you really need to address this phobia first, even if your child is reluctant to.

Once you've chosen which phobia to begin with, you and your child will need to develop a fear list for it. The fear list should contain ten very specific situations that cause increasing levels of anxiety, beginning with ones that elicit only a very little bit of fear all the way up to those that generate a tremendous amount of fear. Use the guidelines, fear scale, and form in Chapter 4 on pages 105–108 to create your child's list. (Extra copies of the form are at the back of the book.)

Remember Evangeline, the eight-year-old who has a phobia of dogs? She and her mom created a fear list. This is what they came up with:

Evangeline's Fear List

Item 1   _Look at an outline of a dog in your coloring book._

Item 2   _Look at a cartoon drawing of a dog in your Highlights magazine._

Item 3   _Look at a photograph of your best friend's dog._

Item 4   _Watch the movie Lassie._

Item 5   _Go to the pet store and look at a puppy in its cage._

Item 6   _Go to the pet store and hold the puppy for one minute._

Item 7   _Go to the pet store and hold/play with the puppy for five minutes._

Item 8   _Go to your best friend's house and look at her dog while it's leashed._

Item 9   _Pet your best friend's dog for one minute._

Item 10   _Hold/play with your best friend's dog for five minutes._

Now that the fear list is in place, Evangeline can start off by working on the first situation (item 1), the easiest one. Once she's done this a number of times and is completely comfortable with it, she can move on the next situation (item 2), which is just a bit harder. One by one, using the same approach, Evangeline will tackle each of the items on her fear list until the final one (item 10) is completed.

With graduated exposure, it's essential that children don't move on to more difficult situations before they're ready to.

Just like Evangeline, your child will need to confront each situation on his or her own fear list. When working on an item, try to arrange for your child to have as many opportunities as possible in the situation. It's also important to have the exposures occur as close together in time as possible. For example, doing three exposure sessions in a week is better than spacing them out over a longer period of time.

When your child faces the same exact situation repeatedly, it eventually will no longer cause anxiety and your child can then move on to the next step. Although I know I've said this before, I want to remind you again that it's *essential* that children *not* move on to a more difficult situation—the next item on the fear list—*until* they are completely comfortable with the one they're currently working on. If they move on to a more difficult task prematurely, there is a risk that the phobia will worsen instead of getting better (this happens through a process called "sensitization," which I talked about previously in Chapter 4).

By the time Evangeline was finished with all the items on her fear list, her phobia of dogs was much better. In fact today she's doing so well that she's been pleading with her mom to get a puppy!

Of all the psychological techniques available for dealing with phobias, there's no question that graduated exposure is the number-one key ingredient to overcoming this anxiety disorder. If you follow the guidelines I've laid out, your child can have the same kind of success that Evangeline did using graduated exposure.

3. Use the imaginal approach to exposure if it's appropriate for your child.

Many phobias—like Evangeline's—involve objects and situations that are encountered (or can be encountered, with a little planning) very frequently, possibly even every day. Other phobias, though, aren't like this. They involve things or circumstances that kids don't run into that often—like flying in a plane or going to the doctor—or are out of our (and all human beings') control—like thunderstorms or facing illness. In cases like this it may not be possible (or desirable—you certainly wouldn't want to create situations to intentionally make your child ill) to use the graduated exposure method I've just described.

When "live" exposure isn't an option, the imaginal method of exposure should be used. The procedure essentially uses the same approach and works the same way as the live version except that the exposure is done in your child's imagination rather than in the real world.

> **Use imaginal exposure when "live" exposure isn't feasible.**

To use the imaginal method, you'll need to come up with the same type of fear list described in the last section (ten very specific situations ranging from ones that cause very minimal levels of anxiety to those that cause extremely high levels of fear). Also, to do exposure through imagination children will need to be in a quiet place where they can recline and close their eyes (the bedroom usually works well for this). They also should be in comfortable clothing (shoes off is best) and have their glasses off if they wear them.

Beginning with the first item (the easiest one), have your child imagine the situation for about a minute. You'll then need to repeat this as many times as it takes for your child to stop experiencing fear or anxiety. Unlike exposure done in the real world, where sessions typically occur on different days, with the imaginal approach you can have multiple exposures occur on the same day, even virtually back to back, as long as you allow a few minutes between them.

Just like with the real-life exposure technique, once your child no longer has any fear or anxiety imagining a situation from the fear list, you can move on to the next item. Again, please remember not to move to the next item until you're sure the one your child currently is working on is no longer a problem. And if you find that the next item on the list is harder for your child than what either of you anticipated (the anxiety is higher than what was expected and/or doesn't seem to be decreasing with repeated exposures), it's a good idea to come up with an "intermediate" step, a situation not quite as difficult as the one your child has just been attempting, but still a bit harder than the one that was just completed successfully.

Do you recall Ali—the eleven-year-old with the phobia of thunderstorms? Because it wasn't feasible to use the live exposure method (since it's not possible to prearrange weather conditions), she and her mom used the imaginal approach to try to get her over her fear. After starting with a situation that caused only a very little bit of anxiety (imagining a cloudy day), Ali was able to take on the rest of the items on her fear list relatively quickly. Not only did she become comfortable picturing the situations; the comfort she achieved in her imagination spilled over to live situations—thunderstorms actually occurring in the *real* world. After just a few short weeks of imaginal exposure, Ali's fear of thunderstorms was gone for good.

Before you decide to proceed with imaginal exposure, I think it's worth knowing that some therapists prefer to do imaginal exposure in combination with a relaxation technique, usually deep muscle relaxation (see Chapter 5, pages 138–140, for a detailed description of how this procedure's done). The idea here is that the relaxation response created by the deep muscle relaxation "competes" with and replaces the anxiety triggered by imagining fearful situations, helping to make the procedure more effective.

Research has shown that the imaginal method is actually just as effective without using deep muscle relaxation, but if you want to spend the time teaching this relaxation method to your child and then use it in conjunction with imaginal exposure, you should go right ahead and do so. Deep muscle relaxation is a very good coping skill for anxious children to learn (I'll be talking more about this later on), and it won't harm your child's chances of succeeding with imaginal exposure. If you decide to use it, however, make sure your child is adept at doing deep muscle relaxation *before* embarking on imaginal exposure. When you begin the exposure sessions, have your child use the deep muscle relaxation right before imagining items from the fear list and then ask him or her to try to maintain the relaxed state throughout the imagery period.

Before we leave the topic of imaginal exposure, I want to tell you about one other circumstance where its use often is appropriate and helpful. We've already discussed the value of using imaginal exposure when it's not feasible to do real-life exposure. But sometimes, even if it is feasible to use live exposure, it may not be the best way to go. Let's take a look at Porsha, a fourth grader with a phobia of elevators, so you can see what I mean.

Porsha and her mom created a fear list and were all set to do the live version of graduated exposure. But when it came to actually working on the first item on the list—just stepping quickly in and out of an elevator while her mom held the "open" button down—Porsha went into a panic, refusing to do it or to try it ever again. Since neither she nor her mom could come up with an item that might be easier to do, they decided to switch to the imaginal exposure approach. Although Porsha couldn't do the fear steps in real life, she was able to conquer them in her imagination. Once this happened, she was able to take on a real elevator using the same items from the fear list, one at a time. For Porsha, imaginal exposure served as a (necessary) prelude to live exposure.

If you find your child isn't able to confront the first item on his or her fear list—and you can't think of a situation that would be less anxiety producing—consider using imaginal exposure, either by itself or, as Porsha and her mom did, as a "lead in" to live exposure.

You might wonder why Porsha's success with imaginal exposure didn't automatically transfer to real-life situations as it had for Ali. While some kids experience a carryover effect, others don't. Unfortunately there's no way to predict which will be the case for your child, so you'll have to see firsthand. If success in imagination doesn't automatically generalize to live situations, go ahead and use the approach that Porsha and her mom used. There's no downside to doing exposure this way (except that it takes a bit longer because situations are tackled twice, first in imagination, then in the real world), and for some kids it's the only approach that will be effective.

4. Teach your child how to get rid of fearful thoughts.

- Ten-year-old Naomi, who has an elevator phobia, is terrified she'll get trapped in one.
- Carmine, a sixth grader with a phobia of flying, is certain the plane will crash.

- Nine-year-old Jane also has a fear of flying, but, unlike Carmine, she doesn't worry about crashing. Her fear is that the plane will "run out of air."
- Harris, a third grader with a height phobia, is scared he's going to fall and get hurt really badly.
- Sabrina, a six-year-old with a phobia of dogs, is petrified she's going to get bitten.

As we talked about in the first chapter in this book, one of the three ways that anxiety and fear express themselves is through thoughts (the other two ways, as you'll recall, are through feelings and behavior). Almost all kids with specific phobias—like the ones I just mentioned—have upsetting, often catastrophic, thoughts about the objects and situations they fear. But although these kinds of thoughts are automatic "by-products" of fear, once they occur they end up *further* increasing anxiety. Not only does this make children even more uncomfortable when faced with the sources of their phobias, it motivates them to escape or avoid these situations, which, in turn, prevents them from getting better.

I think you can see how getting rid of fearful thinking can play a big part in overcoming phobias. But before your child can get rid of these types of thoughts, he or she will need to be aware of them as they are happening. We've discussed this before in Chapters 4 and 7, when talking about separation anxiety and social anxiety disorders. But let's briefly review it again now.

Some kids, like the ones I talked about at the beginning of this section, are acutely aware of their fearful thoughts as they are happening and are readily able to specify what they are and share them with others (which they usually do with their parents, or a therapist if they are receiving professional help). Other children, though, are not as conscious of their thoughts and need help to become aware of them.

If this is the case for your child, there are several ways you can go about doing this. The first, and easiest, is to point out to your child the upsetting, fearful thoughts he or she says out loud in your presence (assuming your child does this), so they become more salient. Another approach is to have kids close their eyes and imagine an actual encounter they've had (preferably one that's happened very recently) with the object or situation they are phobic of and then have them share what they are thinking.

A third method that doesn't rely on having a parent present involves having your child identify fearful thoughts when actually confronted with the object or situation that's the source of the phobia. I usually ask kids to carry a very small spiral notebook with them so they can write down their fearful thoughts while they're in the scary situation or *right after* it's over (if it's right away, they usually are still able to recall their thoughts).

You'll generally find that the fearful thoughts children have in relation to their phobias are pretty consistent and usually limited to just a few specific thoughts—or sometimes even to just one. But if your child has more than one phobia (which, as I've said several times before, isn't at all unusual), each will have its own set of thoughts.

Once your child is aware of the fearful thoughts, it's time to move on to developing the new thoughts that will be used to replace them. The form on the next page can be used to do this. (Please note that the form is to be used for a single phobia, so if your child has more than one phobia, go ahead and make copies of the form and use a separate one for each fear.)

First, at the very top of the form, have your child describe, in his or her own words, the phobia. Then, on the left side of the page, in the area provided for this purpose, have your child write in each of the fearful thoughts, anywhere from one to three of them. Next, directly across from the first fearful thought, on the right side of the paper, ask your child to come up with one or more alternative, positive thoughts (up to three) that can be used to counter or replace the upsetting one. The same, then, should be done with each of the remaining fearful thoughts, assuming your child has more than one (again, as I said before, it's not atypical for kids to have only one fearful thought in relation to a phobia, so don't be concerned if this is the case for your child).

No one can tell you the particular thoughts that will be most effective for your child. Almost always it's the children themselves who are the best judges of how well new thoughts will work at competing with/replacing the old fearful ones. However, it's certainly okay, and can be very helpful, for parents to throw out some ideas

Replacing Scary Thoughts

I'm afraid of _____

My scary thoughts are: *Better thoughts are:*

First scary thought:

_____   1. _____

_____   _____

                                     2. _____

                                     _____

                                     3. _____

                                     _____

Second scary thought:

_____   1. _____

_____   _____

                                     2. _____

                                     _____

                                     3. _____

                                     _____

Third scary thought:

_____   1. _____

_____   _____

                                     2. _____

                                     _____

                                     3. _____

                                     _____

for new thoughts, especially if their children are having trouble coming up with ones on their own. Kids can then pick and choose from what their folks have offered or use their parents' creations as jumping-off points to elaborate from and make the thoughts their very own.

Some kids find that general, coping-type thoughts like "It will be okay" or "I can handle it" are effective, while others need more specific thoughts that directly counter, compete with, or challenge the content of their fearful thoughts.

As you'll recall, Naomi, the girl with the elevator phobia mentioned earlier, had the fearful thought "I'll get trapped." She wrote this down on the left side of her form, in the area for "scary thoughts." Then, across from this, in the column for "better thoughts," she wrote:

1. Elevators almost never get stuck.
2. If the elevator gets stuck, I can press the red emergency button and help will come.
3. If the elevator gets stuck, someone can call for help on the phone in the elevator or on a cell phone.

Naomi practiced coming back at her fearful thought with her new, better thoughts. At first it seemed a bit awkward, but after a while she got more comfortable doing it. Eventually the new thoughts seemed to occur almost automatically. As her thoughts got better, so did Naomi's phobia. Replacing her catastrophic thought with less fearful, more positive ones reduced her anxiety, making it easier for her to ride in elevators.

In fact, it's a very good idea to have your child use this thought replacement technique in combination with graduated exposure (see method 2 above), both before and during exposure sessions. Like Naomi, your child also should practice replacing his or her thoughts anytime the fearful ones occur.

Looking at Naomi's situation, you might wonder how the thought replacement method differs from the educational approach to dealing with phobias (method 1, above). Aren't Naomi's "better thoughts" really just "the facts"?

Although there is some relationship between the two methods, there also are some important differences. The educational approach assumes that providing children with factual information that refutes misunderstandings or misinformation they have about the objects or situations they fear will change the way they look at things and thereby reduce their fear. There is no direct attempt to change children's thoughts, as there is with the thought replacement technique, although providing new information may certainly end up having this effect on them.

The thought replacement approach, on the other hand, doesn't depend on kids' having incorrect information about the sources of their phobias. Fearful thoughts may or may not reflect misunderstandings. For instance, it isn't inaccurate for a child with a phobia of needles to think that getting an injection will hurt—it's not a misconception that needs to be corrected. It's simply a fearful thought that increases anxiety that the child would be better off replacing with a less upsetting, more positive or coping-type thought. The thought replacement technique is a direct approach to changing thoughts that does just this.

Before moving on, I want to mention the possibility that, even after using all of the thought identification methods outlined earlier, your child may not be able to come up with any fearful thoughts. This is what happened to Jada, a nine-year-old with a phobia of cats. After repeated unsuccessful attempts to get at the thoughts, she told her mom, "I just get really nervous as soon as I see one. I don't have time to have any thoughts!"

Some kids with specific phobias (and adults too) report having automatic, physical reactions to the objects and situations they fear and deny having any fearful or catastrophic thoughts. If this is the situation for your child, skip the thought replacement method and go on to the next section, which describes relaxation techniques. It's likely your child will be more successful using an approach that targets the physical manifestations of fear, rather than thoughts.

5. Show your child how to use relaxation techniques to combat fear.

I've discussed the value of relaxation techniques in conquering fear and anxiety in several of the other chapters in this book. To review again briefly here, relaxation techniques work by decreasing autonomic nervous system activity, which, in turn, can reduce the unpleasant physical feelings that are part of fear and anxiety.

There are two particular relaxation methods that I like to use with children. The first is *deep breathing*, which was discussed at length in Chapter 4 (see pages 111–112 for how to do it). The technique involves teaching kids to breathe more slowly and deeply, from the diaphragm. (When kids are afraid, they tend to hyperventilate—breathe rapidly and shallowly, from the upper chest, which increases feelings of anxiety.) The other method is *deep muscle relaxation*, which was described in detail in Chapter 5 (see pages 138–140 for how this is done) and mentioned earlier in this chapter when I was discussing imaginal exposure (see method 3, above). To summarize, this method of relaxation focuses on reducing muscular tension through a series of exercises that target different areas of the body.

For specific phobias, relaxation techniques are particularly helpful when kids are being exposed to, or anticipating being exposed to, the object or situation they fear. For that reason it's especially good to use a relaxation method (either one, depending on your child's preference) in conjunction with graduated exposure (see method 2, above), just as I suggested for the thought replacement technique too.

> Using the thought replacement technique or a relaxation method in combination with graduated exposure can make the procedure much more effective.

While it's certainly fine to use both a relaxation method and the thought technique during exposure sessions, your child may find that one is more helpful than the other. For instance, kids who are very sensitive to the physical manifestations of fear—butterflies in the stomach, pounding heart, etc.—or those who deny having any fearful or catastrophic thoughts (like Jada, discussed a little while ago), may be better off using a relaxation method, while children who are preoccupied with catastrophic thoughts may benefit more from the thought replacement method.

As you have just seen, the essential measure for overcoming specific phobias is for kids to gradually face the objects and situations they fear, either in the "real world" or in their imagination or with a combination of both approaches. Along with providing educational material to correct any misconceptions your child may have about the source of his or her phobia and thought and relaxation techniques to reduce anxiety, your child now has all the tools needed to overcome this problem.

RESOURCES

If Your Child Needs Professional Help

Evaluation and Treatment Centers

On the next few pages I've listed a number of centers and programs that specialize in evaluating and treating anxiety disorders in children. The list is by no means exhaustive (there are many more places that specialize in this area), but they are the programs (or directors) I've been most familiar with and impressed by during my career.

Please note that the facilities included here are all associated with universities (as opposed to centers or clinics operated by private practitioners). I like to refer families to university-based centers (or directly to faculty affiliated with an educational institution) because places like this usually are "on the cutting edge" in terms of having knowledge about and utilizing the very latest, most effective treatments available for psychiatric and psychological problems. (That's not to say there aren't countless numbers of individuals in private practice who are just as knowledgeable and up to date. I'll be giving you ways to go about locating professionals like this a little later on in this section.)

Some of the programs offer services only to children and families that meet specific research criteria for studies they are conducting (the upside to this is that the services, in these cases, usually are free of charge). Others offer clinical services as part of the training of doctoral students (usually on a sliding fee basis) or from faculty (as part of their clinical responsibilities or as part of a practice plan the university maintains for its faculty).

If you contact one of the sites listed, make sure you find out who will be providing services to your child (a doctoral student supervised by a seasoned mental health professional; a faculty or staff member), whether it will be part of a research project, and what the cost will be to you.

The centers are listed in alphabetical order by state. At the end of the list I've also included a few programs from other English-speaking countries for readers in Canada and abroad.

The UCLA Childhood OCD, Anxiety, and Tic Disorders Program
Los Angeles, CA

Director: John Piacentini, PhD
Telephone: (310) 825-4132 (clinic coordinator)
Website: *www.npi.ucla.edu/caap*

   This clinical and research program specializes in the evaluation and treatment of anxiety and related problems in children and adolescents.

Child Anxiety and Phobia Program
Miami, FL

Director: Wendy K. Silverman, PhD
Telephone: (305) 348-1937 or (305) 348-1938
Website: *www.fiu.edu/~capp*

   The program is conducted at Florida International University with the research support of the National Institute of Mental Health. It provides comprehensive diagnostic assessments and cognitive-behavioral treatment to children and adolescents, ages eight to fourteen, who are experiencing excessive fear- and anxiety-related problems.

The Child and Adolescent Anxiety Treatment Program
Boston, MA

Director: Donna B. Pincus, PhD
Telephone: (617) 353-9610
Website: *www.bu.edu/anxiety/adolescent*

   The program, which is part of Boston University's Center for Anxiety and Related Disorders, offers comprehensive evaluations and cognitive-behavioral treatment to children and adolescents, ages seven to seventeen, who are having problems with fears, anxiety, or shyness.

Child and Adolescent Anxiety and Mood Disorders Clinic
Minneapolis, MN

Director: Gail A. Bernstein, MD
Telephone: (612) 273-8710

   The clinic, located at the University of Minnesota Medical School, provides diagnostic evaluations, cognitive-behavioral therapy, and medication management to children and adolescents with anxiety or mood disorders.

Anxiety Disorders Center at Saint Louis University School of Medicine
St. Louis, MO

Director: C. Alec Pollard, PhD

Telephone: (314) 534-0200
E-mail: info@slbmi.com
Website: *www.slbmi.com*

The Anxiety Disorders Center, as part of the Saint Louis Behavioral Medicine Institute, provides assessment and treatment services (therapy and medication) to children and adults who have anxiety disorders. In addition to standard outpatient treatment, the center offers intensive outpatient treatment, partial hospitalization, home-based care, and a special program for "difficult-to-treat" cases.

University of Nevada, Las Vegas, Child School Refusal and Anxiety Disorders Clinic

Las Vegas, NV
Director: Christopher A. Kearney, PhD
Telephone: (702) 895-0183
E-mail: ckearney@ccmail.nevada.edu

The clinic provides assessment and treatment services to youths ages five to fifteen who have school refusal behavior and/or anxiety disorders. The clinic is a nonprofit agency on the UNLV campus that provides services based on a family's ability to pay.

Child Anxiety Disorders Clinic

Hackensack, NJ
Director: Andrew R. Eisen, PhD
Telephone: (201) 692-2593
E-mail: eisen@fdu.edu
Website: *www.fdu.edu/centers/cps/cadc*

The Child Anxiety Disorders Clinic is a clinical and research specialty clinic of Fairleigh Dickinson University's Center for Psychological Services. It specializes in the cognitive-behavioral assessment and treatment of anxiety and related disorders in children and adolescents, ages three to seventeen.

Columbia University Center for Anxiety Disorders

New York, NY
Director: Anne Marie Albano, PhD
Telephone: (212) 543-5339

The center specializes in consultation, diagnostic evaluation, and cognitive-behavioral therapy for children, adolescents, and young adults with anxiety disorders.

Duke Program in Child Anxiety and Affective Disorders
Durham, NC
Director: John S. March, MD
Telephone: (919) 416-7200
E-mail: psychinfo@mc.duke.edu
Website: *www.mentalhealth.dukehealth.org*
    The program offers diagnostic evaluations and treatment—cognitive-behavioral therapy, family therapy, and medication—for children and adolescents with anxiety or mood disorders.

Child and Adolescent Anxiety Disorders Clinic
Philadelphia, PA
Director: Philip C. Kendall, PhD
Telephone: (215) 204-7165
Website: *www.childanxiety.org*
    The clinic, located at Temple University, specializes in providing services to children and adolescents, ages seven to seventeen, who suffer from anxiety problems. The program is particularly well known for its use of the "Coping Cat" approach, a cognitive-behavioral treatment for kids seven to thirteen with generalized anxiety disorder, separation anxiety disorder, or specific phobias (Dr. Kendall is the originator of this treatment approach).

Anxiety Clinic for Children and Adolescents at the University of Pittsburgh School of Medicine
Pittsburgh, PA
Director: Boris Birmaher, MD
Telephone: (412) 246-5606
E-mail: harmonhn@upmc.edu (clinic coordinator)
    The anxiety clinic is part of the Services for Teens at Risk and specializes in the assessment and treatment (cognitive-behavioral therapy and medication) of children and adolescents, ages six to eighteen, with generalized anxiety disorder, separation anxiety disorder, and specific phobias.

Child Anxiety Projects at Virginia Polytechnic Institute and State University
Blacksburg, VA
Director: Thomas H. Ollendick, PhD
Telephone: (540) 231-6451
E-mail: tho@vt.edu
    Three different projects offer treatment services as part of large-scale

government-funded research studies for children and adolescents ages seven to sixteen who have specific phobias, social phobia, or school refusal (school phobia).

Outside the United States

The Macquarie University Anxiety Unit
Sydney, Australia
Director: Ron Rapee, PhD
Telephone: (02) 9850-8711
E-mail: muaru@psy.mq.edu.au
Website: *www.psy.mq.edu.au/MUARU*

The clinic runs group treatment programs for clinically anxious children and adolescents (called Cool Kids) and also has an outreach program for more rural and remote areas of Australia.

Anxiety Clinic of the Department of Child Psychiatry of McGill University
Montreal, Canada
Director: Klaus Minde, MD, FRCP(C)
Telephone: (514) 412-4449
E-mail: klaus.minde@mcgill.ca

This clinic, located at Montreal Children's Hospital, offers treatment services (cognitive-behavioral therapy and other types of psychotherapy, as well as medication) to anxious children ages two to eleven.

Child Anxiety Programs at the University of Montreal
Montreal, Canada
Director: Lyse Turgeon, PhD
Telephone: (514) 251-4015, ext. 2362

Three programs are being conducted at the Louis-H. Lafontaine Hospital: one for school-age children with anxiety problems in general, one specifically for children with PTSD, and one for anxious parents to prevent the development of anxiety problems in their school-age children. I am told that in September of 2005 a new clinic will open for children with anxiety disorders at Riviere-des-Prairies Hospital in Montreal, also affiliated with the University of Montreal.

Anxiety Disorders Team at the Hospital for Sick Children
Toronto, Canada
Director: Katharina Manassis, MD, FRCPC

Telephone: (416) 813-6582
E-mail: veronica.romano@sickkids.ca (intake coordinator)
Website: *www.sickkids.ca/psychiatry*

This anxiety center, which is affiliated with the Department of Psychiatry at the University of Toronto, is a clinical research program offering consultation, assessment, and treatment (cognitive-behavioral and medication interventions) for anxious children ages five to seventeen. The center is quite large and well respected by professionals in Canada, and other countries too, who specialize in childhood anxiety disorders.

Anxiety Disorders Research Clinic at the University of Reading
Reading, England
Director: Dr. Tim Williams (clinical) and Prof. Peter Cooper
  (research)
Telephone: (0) 118 931 5880

The clinic offers assessment and treatment services for children and adolescents with anxiety disorders who live in Berkshire County.

Berkshire OCD Clinic
Wokingham, England
Director: Dr. Tim Williams
Telephone: (0) 118 949 5019

This clinic, which is affiliated with the University of Reading, offers treatment services for children and adolescents with obsessive–compulsive disorder who live in Berkshire County.

Websites Where You Can Locate Individual Practitioners

Here are a few websites that include provider lists that can help you find a mental health professional for your child in your own geographical area. I've included telephone numbers as well as the website addresses in case you don't have access to the Internet or just prefer to call. Most of these websites offer a good deal of information about anxiety disorders so they can be helpful in this respect too.

American Academy of Child and Adolescent Psychiatry
www.aacap.org
Telephone: (202) 966-7300

The AACAP is a professional organization that consists of physicians who specialize in child and adolescent psychiatry. In addition to containing a referral directory so you can find a child psychiatrist in your area, the site has good information on how to go about choosing a child psychiatrist. Surprisingly, for a very-high-level professional organization, this website is extremely parent-friendly.

Anxiety Disorders Association of America
www.adaa.org
Telephone: (240) 485-1001

The ADAA is a large organization that has both professional and nonprofessional members. The provider list on this site is extensive, as it includes most of ADAA's professional members, and it's in alphabetical order by state (it also includes providers in other countries, but primarily Canada, with thirty-eight listings at the present time). All of the providers—psychologists, psychiatrists, social workers, and other types of mental health professionals—treat anxiety disorders, but not all treat children. You'll have to read the individual profiles (which are included for everyone on the list) of practitioners to see whether or not they offer services to kids.

Association for Behavioral and Cognitive Therapies
www.aabt.org
Telephone: (212) 647-1890

This large organization just recently changed its name. However, the Web address and website still, at the time I'm writing this, use the old name—*Association for Advancement of Behavior Therapy* (AABT). The organization includes professional members only (mostly psychologists), who have a behavioral or cognitive-behavioral orientation, and has a referral list of therapists that consists of their members who have private practices. The way you search for a therapist on this site allows for a great deal of specificity (age group, problem, type of treatment you're looking for), so you're likely to find just what you're looking for.

Child Anxiety Network
www.childanxiety.net
Telephone: (617) 353-9610

This website was developed by Dr. Donna Pincus, who also is the director of Boston University's Child and Adolescent Anxiety Treatment Program (see page 242). The provider list on this site includes mental health professionals, mostly psychologists, who specialize in treating childhood anxiety disorders.

Cognitive Therapy Center of Brooklyn
www.cognitivetherapy.com
Telephone: (718) 636-5071 (voicemail box 1)

This website was created by John Winston Bush, PhD, who is the director of Brooklyn's center for cognitive therapy (Dr. Bush's private practice). This site can be helpful in finding a cognitive-behavioral therapist in your own geographical area, but you'll have to contact the provider yourself to find out if he or she works with kids and specializes in treating anxiety disorders in this age group. The site also answers questions about cognitive therapy (for example, "What is cognitive-behavior therapy?") so you can become more familiar with what constitutes this treatment approach.

Obsessive–Compulsive Foundation
www.ocfoundation.org
Telephone: (203) 401-2070

This foundation, as the name implies, focuses exclusively on obsessive–compulsive disorder. It is very well known and has an excellent reputation among professionals who specialize in this area, as well as "consumers" (people who have OCD). In addition to having a "mental health referral list," the site contains a wealth of information on OCD, including information about the disorder in children.

Outside the United States

The British Association for Behavioural and Cognitive Psychotherapies
www.babcp.com
Telephone: (0) 125 487 5277

This website has an extensive list of cognitive-behavioral practitioners throughout the United Kingdom. You can search for one by location, the age group you're interested in (for our purposes here, "children and adolescence"), and problem area (for instance, "anxiety/panic attacks" or "obsessive–compulsive disorder").

Associations and Organizations

Many of the websites listed above provide a wealth of information on mental health issues and problems as well as helping you find a doctor for your child (if your son or daughter needs professional help.) The associations and organizations listed here do not provide direct referrals (some of them, though, have "links" to other sites that do this), but they do contain information that is quite valuable.

American Psychiatric Association
Washington, DC
Telephone: (703) 907-7300 or (888) 357-7924
E-mail: apa@psych.org
Website: *www.psych.org*

This is the largest professional organization for psychiatrists in the United States. The website contains a great deal of information for the public, including guidelines on how to choose a psychiatrist.

American Psychological Association
Washington, DC
Telephone: (202) 336-5500 or (800) 374-2721
Website: *www.apa.org*

The American Psychological Association is the largest professional association for psychologists in the United States. The website's "Help Center" is an online resource for brochures, tips, and articles on mental health issues, including anxiety disorders.

National Institute of Mental Health
Bethesda, MD
Telephone: (301) 443-4513
Website: *www.nimh.nih.gov*

The NIMH, which is part of the National Institutes of Health (NIH), is a national government agency that sponsors research and disseminates the results of these studies to other professionals and the public at large. This is an especially good website to visit to get the very latest information on childhood anxiety disorders from a scientific perspective.

Outside the United States

Royal Australian and New Zealand College of Psychiatrists
Melbourne, Australia
Telephone: 61-3-9640-0646
E-mail: ranzcp@ranzcp.org
Website: *www.ranzcp.org*

The college is the main body representing psychiatry in Australia and New Zealand, with over 2,500 "fellows." The website contains a range of information about psychiatry in these countries, as well as links to sites that contain even more information about mental health, including anxiety disorders.

Anxiety Disorders Alliance
New South Wales, Australia
Telephone: (02) 9816-2826
E-mail: ada@ada.mentalhealth.asn.au
Website: *www.ada.mentalhealth.asn.au*

The ADA primarily is an information service for children and adults who have anxiety problems. The alliance also has initiated a program called "Small Steps," which is for parents and teachers of primary-school-age children (kindergarten through sixth grade) with anxiety disorders. The program consists of two components: information seminars conducted for teachers and parents, and support groups for parents of children who have anxiety disorders. To get in touch with the Small Steps project you can call or e-mail using the information above.

Canadian Psychiatric Association
Ottawa, Ontario, Canada
Telephone: (613) 234-2815
E-mail: cpa@cpa-apc.org
Website: *www.cpa-apc.org*

This is Canada's national professional association for psychiatrists, similar to the *American Psychiatric Association* in the United States. Although the website does not contain a referral list, it addresses important issues facing both adult and child psychiatry. The association contains three "academies," one of which is the Canadian Academy of Child and Adolescent Psychiatry.

Canadian Psychological Association
Ottawa, Ontario, Canada
Telephone: (613) 237-2144
Website: *www.cpa.ca*

This is the national association for psychologists in Canada. The website primarily is intended for psychologists (and other mental health professionals) with the exception of the section entitled "Psychology Works" (which was prepared by the clinical division of the association). It contains in-depth information on a wide range of psychological/psychiatric problems, including anxiety disorders.

Anxiety Disorders Association of Canada
Scarborough, Ontario, Canada
Telephone: (888) 223-2252 (toll free)
E-mail: contactus@anxietycanada.ca
Website: *www.anxietycanada.ca*

A Canadian colleague of mine referred to this association as "the little sister to the *Anxiety Disorders Association of America*" (see page 247). The website has a wealth of information on anxiety disorders, including in children, but does not contain a list of providers (the ADAA one does and, in fact, a number of Canadians are included on it). In total, there are four provincial ADAC associations across Canada. In addition to the one listed here, the other three are in British Columbia, Quebec, and Manitoba. You can get their contact information directly off the website address I gave you above.

The Royal College of Psychiatrists
London, United Kingdom
Telephone: 020 7235 2351
Website: *www.rcpsych.ac.uk*

The website for the college has a section entitled "Mental Health Information" that consumers can click on and then fine-tune their search by the type of problem they're interested in learning more about (for example, "Anxiety and Phobias"; "Obsessive Compulsive Disorder") and/or the age group they're inquiring about ("Young People" or "Older People"). Although the national headquarters of the college is in London, there are regional divisions in Ireland (Dublin), Northern Ireland (Belfast), Scotland (Edinburgh), and Wales (Cardiff). Contact information for the regional divisions is on the website.

Books

A great many books have been written for adults who have anxiety disorders, but, as I indicated in the preface of this book, very few for parents who have children with these problems. There are, though, many story books that deal with the issues that face anxious kids. The few I've included here were selected because they've proven to be the most helpful to the families I work with. It's a good idea to read them together with your child.

The Good-Bye Book by Judith Viorst, Macmillan Publishing Company, 1988.

This book is excellent for young kids who have problems with separation anxiety. Although no age group is specified, I'd say it's appropriate for children ages four through seven.

The Runaway Bunny by Margaret Wise Brown, Harper & Row, 1970.

This book is "a classic"—it was first published in 1942 and since then has never been out of print. It was written for kids ages three through seven and is especially good for children who have separation anxiety but also may be helpful for boys and girls with other types of anxiety problems. (As an aside, this book is really beautifully illustrated!)

Blink, Blink, Clop, Clop: Why Do We Do Things We Can't Stop? An OCD Storybook by E. Katia Moritz and Jennifer Jablonsky, Childwork/Childsplay of Genesis Direct, Inc., 1998. (This book must be ordered directly from the publisher by calling toll free: 1-800-962-1141.)

This "OCD Storybook" was developed specifically for young children who have obsessive–compulsive disorder. The first author—Dr. Moritz—is a child psychologist who specializes in this area. The book is appropriate for kids ages four through eight.

As I've discussed in several places in this book, it's not unusual for parents of anxious children to have anxiety problems themselves. Below are several self-help books that I've found to be outstanding at giving adults specific, concrete skills they can use to combat anxiety disorders.

The Anxiety and Phobia Workbook (third edition) by Edmund J. Bourne, PhD, New Harbinger Publications, 2000 (paperback).

Don't Panic: Taking Control of Anxiety Attacks (revised edition) by R. Reid Wilson, PhD, HarperCollins, 1996 (paperback).

The Hidden Face of Shyness: Understanding & Overcoming Social Anxiety (revised edition) by Franklin Schneier, MD, and Lawrence Welkowitz, PhD, Avon Books, 1996 (paperback).

Stop Obsessing!: How to Overcome Your Obsessions and Compulsions (revised edition) by Edna B. Foa, PhD, and R. Reid Wilson, PhD, Bantam Books, 2001 (paperback).

If you are working with a therapist to address an anxiety problem of your own, I highly recommend Dr. David H. Barlow's treatment manuals: *Mastering Your Anxiety and Panic* (for panic attacks and panic disorder) and *Mastering Your Anxiety and Worry* (for generalized anxiety disorder). There are separate client and therapist manuals, both of which are available from Oxford University Press (*www.oup.com*).

Although I haven't read this book (it's on my "to do" list), many of my adult patients who have OCD have recommended it to me:

Brain Lock: Free Yourself from Obsessive–Compulsive Behavior by Jeffrey M. Schwartz, MD, Regan Books, 1997.

If you or your child has obsessive–compulsive disorder, I strongly recommend:

The Boy Who Couldn't Stop Washing: The Experience and Treatment of Obsessive–Compulsive Disorder by Judith L. Rapoport, MD, Penguin Books, 1991 (paperback).

Dr. Rapoport has brought her many years of research and clinical experience to bear in shedding light on this very complex disorder. Even though the book was written a while ago, it remains, in my opinion, one of the very best on this subject.

How to Contact Me

I have offices located in Boca Raton and Delray Beach, Florida. To contact me by mail you can use the following address:

Dr. Cynthia G. Last
110 S. E. 4th Ave, Suite 106
Delray Beach, FL 33483

By telephone you can call me at (561) 272-4941 (Delray Beach) or (561) 852-5886 (Boca Raton).

If you wish to e-mail me, you can write to either of these addresses:

CGLast@aol.com
CGLast@bellsouth.net

I look forward to hearing from you!

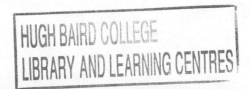

CHECKLISTS AND WORKSHEETS

Extra copies of some of the forms that appear throughout this book are contained in the pages that follow.

The Child Anxiety Checklist

Does your child . . .	Yes	No
Have recurrent stomachaches or headaches, for which there is no medical cause?	☐	☐
Have fears that are excessive (more intense than those of other children of similar age) or inappropriate for his or her age?	☐	☐
Have "nervous habits," such as nail biting, "restless legs," knuckle cracking, playing with hair, etc.?	☐	☐
Worry a lot? About a lot of different things?	☐	☐
Complain of upsetting thoughts or pictures (mental images)?	☐	☐
Engage in repetitive behaviors that must be performed but don't "make sense"?	☐	☐
Appear overly concerned or perfectionistic about performance in certain activities, either in or outside of school?	☐	☐
Exhibit anxiety when in social situations or when he or she is the center of attention?	☐	☐
Have trouble making friends because of excessive shyness?	☐	☐
Have frequent nightmares or bad dreams?	☐	☐
Tend to avoid or run away from frightening, but not dangerous, things (as opposed to confronting the feared object or situation)?	☐	☐
Get nervous in new situations or unfamiliar places?	☐	☐
Have a history of experiencing or witnessing a traumatic event, one that threatened his or her own, or someone else's, physical well-being?	☐	☐
Need a lot of reassurance?	☐	☐
Have trouble with changes in routine or a change in plans?	☐	☐

Child Anxiety Checklist Ratings

Checklist item (describe)	Ratings ("1," "2," or "3")	
	Distress	Functioning
_____	_____	_____
_____	_____	_____
_____	_____	_____
_____	_____	_____
_____	_____	_____
_____	_____	_____
_____	_____	_____
_____	_____	_____

My Worries: Better Ways to Look at Things

What I'm worried will happen:

_____

_____

_____

_____

Other ways to think about it:

1. _____

_____

_____

_____

2. _____

_____

_____

_____

3. _____

_____

_____

_____

My Worries: Better Ways to Look at Things

What I'm worried will happen:

_____

_____

_____

_____

Other ways to think about it:

1. _____

_____

_____

_____

2. _____

_____

_____

_____

3. _____

_____

_____

_____

My Worries: Better Ways to Look at Things

What I'm worried will happen:

_____

_____

_____

_____

Other ways to think about it:

1. _____

_____

_____

_____

2. _____

_____

_____

_____

_____

3. _____

_____

_____

_____

Weekly Record

Monday

_____

_____

Tuesday

_____

_____

Wednesday

_____

_____

Thursday

_____

_____

Friday

_____

_____

Saturday

_____

_____

Sunday

_____

_____

Weekly Record

Monday

_____

_____

Tuesday

_____

_____

Wednesday

_____

_____

Thursday

_____

_____

Friday

_____

_____

Saturday

_____

_____

Sunday

_____

_____

Weekly Record

Monday

_____

_____

Tuesday

_____

_____

Wednesday

_____

_____

Thursday

_____

_____

Friday

_____

_____

Saturday

_____

_____

Sunday

_____

_____

Your Child's Fear List

Item 1 (the easiest situation)

_____

Item 2

_____

Item 3

_____

Item 4

_____

Item 5

_____

Item 6

_____

Item 7

_____

Item 8

_____

Item 9

_____

Item 10 (the hardest situation)

_____

SELECTED SCIENTIFIC ARTICLES BY THE AUTHOR

Much of the information and advice in this book is based on my research. Readers who are interested in more detail will find the data in the following articles (in chronological order).

Last CG, Francis G, Hersen M, Kazdin AE, & Strauss CC: Separation anxiety and school phobia: A comparison using DSM-III criteria. *American Journal of Psychiatry,* **144**: 653–657, 1987.

Last CG, Hersen M, Kazdin AE, Finkelstein R, & Strauss CC: Comparison of DSM-III separation anxiety and overanxious disorders: Demographic characteristics and patterns of comorbidity. *Journal of the American Academy of Child and Adolescent Psychiatry,* **26**: 527–531, 1987.

Last CG, Strauss CC, & Francis G: Cormobidity among childhood anxiety disorders. *Journal of Nervous and Mental Disease,* **175**: 726–730, 1987.

Francis G, **Last** CG, & Strauss CC: Expression of separation anxiety disorder: The roles of age and gender. *Child Psychiatry and Human Development,* **18**: 82–89, 1987.

Strauss CC, **Last** CG, Hersen M, & Kazdin AE: Association between anxiety and depression in children and adolescents with anxiety disorders. *Journal of Abnormal Child Psychology,* **15**: 57–68, 1988.

Strauss CC, Lease CL, **Last** CG, & Francis G: Overanxious disorder: An examination of developmental differences. *Journal of Abnormal Child Psychology,* **16**: 433–443, 1988.

Last CG, & Strauss CC: Panic disorder in children and adolescents. *Journal of Anxiety Disorders,* **3**: 87–95, 1989.

Last CG, Francis G, & Strauss CC: Assessing fears in anxiety disordered children with the Revised Fear Survey Schedule for Children (FSSC-R). *Journal of Clinical Child Psychology,* **18**: 137–141, 1989.

Strauss CC, Lease CA, Kazdin AE, Dulcan MK, & **Last** CG: Multimethod assessment of the social competence of children with anxiety disorders. *Journal of Clinical Child Psychology,* **18**: 184–189, 1989.

Last CG, & Strauss CC: Obsessive–compulsive disorder in childhood. *Journal of Anxiety Disorders,* **3**: 295–302, 1989.

Last CG, & Strauss CC: School refusal in anxiety disordered children and adolescents. *Journal of the American Academy of Child and Adolescent Psychiatry*, **29**: 31–35, 1990.

Bell-Dolan DJ, Last CG, & Strauss CC: Symptoms of anxiety disorders in normal children. *Journal of the American Academy of Child and Adolescent Psychiatry*, **29**: 759–765, 1990.

Last CG, Hersen M, Kazdin AE, Orvaschel H, & Perrin S: Anxiety disorders in children and their families. *Archives of General Psychiatry* **48**: 928–934.

Last, CG: Somatic complaints in anxiety disordered children. *Journal of Anxiety Disorders*, **5**: 125–138, 1991.

Last CG, Perrin S, Hersen M, & Kazdin AE: DSM-III-R anxiety disorders in children: Sociodemographic and clinical characteristics. *Journal of the American Academy of Child and Adolescent Psychiatry*, **31**: 1070–1076, 1992.

Strauss CC, & Last CG: Social and simple phobias in children. *Journal of Anxiety Disorders*, **7**: 141–152, 1993.

Last CG, Perrin S, Hersen M, Kazdin AE: A prospective study of childhood anxiety disorders. *Journal of the American Academy of Child and Adolescent Psychiatry*, **35**: 1502–1510, 1996.

Perrin S, & Last CG: Relationship between ADHD and anxiety in boys: Results from a family study. *Journal of the American Academy of Child and Adolescent Psychiatry*, **35**: 988–996, 1996.

Perrin S, & Last CG: Worrisome thoughts in children clinically referred for anxiety disorders. *Journal of Clinical Child Psychology*, **26**: 181–189, 1997.

Last CG, Hansen C, & Franco N: Anxious children in adulthood: A prospective study of adjustment. *Journal of the American Academy of Child and Adolescent Psychiatry*, **36**: 637–652, 1997.

Hansen C, Levinson L, & Last CG: "Correspondence between DSM-III-R OAD and DSM-IV GAD in Clinically-Referred Children and Adolescents." Paper presented at the First Annual Conference on Assessment Psychology, Orlando, FL, April 1998.

Last CG, Hansen C, & Franco N: Cognitive-behavioral treatment of school phobia. *Journal of the American Academy of Child and Adolescent Psychiatry*, **37**: 404–411, 1998.

Bernstein G, Borchardt C, Perwien AR, Crosby RD, Kushner MG, Thuras PD, & Last CG: Imipramine plus cognitive-behavioral therapy in the treatment of school refusal. *Journal of the American Academy of Child and Adolescent Psychiatry*, **39**: 276–283, 2000.

INDEX

ABOUT THE AUTHOR

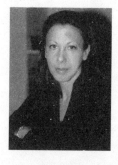

Cynthia G. Last, PhD, is recognized internationally as a leading expert on childhood fears and anxiety. She has been the recipient of numerous research grants from the National Institute of Mental Health to study fears and anxiety in children, and she served as an advisor to the American Psychiatric Association on modifying the child anxiety section of the third (revised) and fourth editions of the *Diagnostic and Statistical Manual of Mental Disorders,* the diagnostic classification system used in the United States and abroad.

Dr. Last is the author or editor of twelve books on anxiety and/or child psychiatry. She has taught hundreds of graduate and postgraduate students in psychology and psychiatry, first as Professor of Child Psychiatry at the University of Pittsburgh School of Medicine and later as Professor of Psychology at Nova Southeastern University in Fort Lauderdale, Florida.

In addition to her academic pursuits, Dr. Last has devoted herself to mental health practice. She founded and directed the Child and Adolescent Anxiety Disorder Clinic at the University of Pittsburgh School of Medicine and the Child and Adolescent Anxiety Disorder Program at Nova Southeastern University. She has also maintained her own practice throughout her career, where she specializes in the cognitive-behavioral treatment of anxiety disorders in children, adolescents, and adults.

Dr. Last has received extensive media coverage in the national press, and her reputation as an outstanding therapist gained her inclusion in *Good Housekeeping* magazine's list of "The 327 Best Mental Health Experts" in the United States. She has also appeared on national television and radio programs.